Why Do I Have **Asperger's?**

A Mother's Memoir of Love, Hope, and Perseverance

JULIE BERRY

LUCIDBOOKS

Why Do I Have Asperger's?
A Mother's Memoir of Love, Hope, and Perseverance
Copyright © 2018 by Julie Berry

Published by Lucid Books in Houston, TX
www.LucidBooksPublishing.com

All rights reserved. No part of this publication may be reproduced, stored in a retrieval system, or transmitted in any form by any means, electronic, mechanical, photocopy, recording, or otherwise, without the prior permission of the publisher, except as provided for by USA copyright law.

Unless otherwise indicated, all Scripture quotations are taken from the ESV® Bible (The Holy Bible, English Standard Version®), copyright © 2001 by Crossway, a publishing ministry of Good News Publishers. Used by permission. All rights reserved.

Scripture quotations marked (NIV) are taken from the Holy Bible, New International Version®, NIV®. Copyright ©1973, 1978, 1984, 2011 by Biblica, Inc.™ Used by permission of Zondervan. All rights reserved worldwide. www.zondervan.com The "NIV" and "New International Version" are trademarks registered in the United States Patent and Trademark Office by Biblica, Inc.™

Scripture quotations marked (NLT) are taken from the Holy Bible, New Living Translation, copyright ©1996, 2004, 2007, 2013, 2015 by Tyndale House Foundation. Used by permission of Tyndale House Publishers, Inc., Carol Stream, Illinois 60188. All rights reserved.

Author has changed certain names and locations within these events for privacy purposes.

Lyrics from "Stronger" by Mandisa: Copyright © 2011 Regisfunk Music (BMI) 9t One Songs (ASCAP) Ariose Music (ASCAP) Universal Music Brentwood. Benson Publ. (ASCAP) D Soul Music (ASCAP) (adm. At CapitolCMGPublishing.com) All rights reserved. Used by permission.

 ISBN-10: 1-63296-188-1
 ISBN-13: 978-1-63296-188-4
 eISBN-10: 1-63296-189-X
 eISBN-13: 978-1-63296-189-1

Special Sales: Most Lucid Books titles are available in special quantity discounts. Custom imprinting or excerpting can also be done to fit special needs. Contact Lucid Books at Info@LucidBooksPublishing.com.

I would like to dedicate this book to all the coaches at Behavior Plus who worked with Jacob. To Nancy Kling, Nannette Samson, Jenn Zapata, Tricia DelBello, and Cristi Walters—every one of you is the reason Jacob has had such incredible progress and success since his diagnosis. I truly don't know where we would be today without your patience, expertise, and commitment to my son. Thank you so very much.

Table of Contents

Prologue	vii
1: Before the Diagnosis	1
2: After the Diagnosis	15
3: Help Wanted	31
4: First Steps	35
5: I Will Fight You	49
6: Getting Somewhere	63
7: Leaps and Bounds	85
8: Speak Life	119
Epilogue	125

PROLOGUE

"**M**om, why did God give me Asperger's?" I stepped on the brake. We were pulling out of the garage on the way to Jacob's behavior group. My heart skipped a beat as I fought down a brief feeling of panic. How could I answer that question? How could I reassure this young boy that the God he loves only wants the best for him? How could I help him understand that God always works everything for our good even when it hurts? How could I begin to describe a condition that I was still striving to understand myself? I took a deep breath, gathered my thoughts, and continued to back down the driveway.

Asperger's syndrome is a neurobiological disorder on the higher-functioning end of the autism spectrum. People with Asperger's syndrome are deficient in communication skills and lack the ability to make effective social connections.

According to the Centers for Disease Control, from 2000 to 2012, children diagnosed on the autism spectrum rose from 1 in 150 to a staggering 1 in 68.* As the number of people diagnosed with Asperger's syndrome increases,

---

*"Autism Spectrum Disorder," *Centers for Disease Control and Prevention*, accessed November 25, 2017 at https://www.cdc.gov/ncbddd/autism/data.html.

the lives of thousands of parents, siblings, friends, and teachers are continually impacted.

On numerous occasions, I've had the opportunity to share with others my family's experiences, both good and bad, in dealing with Asperger's syndrome. Every time I've written anything for public consumption through social media or my blog, I've been contacted by friends who ask questions for themselves or seek permission to share my son's story with a relative or friend. This consistent search for answers from people I barely know or have never even met is a major impetus for the writing of this book.

You may be walking through a difficult time or know someone who is. Perhaps you too have just received that diagnosis that causes you to question your core beliefs and ask, "Why does God allow this?"

That is why I want to share our story, a story that includes a frantic search for answers, numerous questions, multiple visits to medical professionals, battles with educators, and years of behavior modification. These are stories of heartache and frustration that, with time, yielded remarkable progress and life-changing achievement.

Jacob was nine when he asked why God gave him Asperger's syndrome, only three years since his diagnosis at the age of six. His name is Jacob Berry. His strength and determination inspire me as a parent, a mom, and a believer. But he hasn't walked this road alone.

1
BEFORE THE DIAGNOSIS

I praise you, for I am fearfully and wonderfully made.
—Psalm 139:14

Welcome to the Family
"When can I see him?"

It had been twenty-four long hours. I delivered my second son, Jacob, by Caesarean section at 10:48 a.m. on a Tuesday in February 1999. I wasn't able to hold him or touch him for a full excruciating day and night. He had low blood sugar and had to be connected to an IV that was attached to his head. Having a nurse bring him to me wasn't going to happen. I was still numb from the waist down due to the spinal I was administered before delivery and was confined to bed with tubes and wires all over my body.

I couldn't sleep. It felt as if a part of me were missing. Every time the hospital door opened, I caught my breath as my heart pounded, thinking that finally I would get to meet Jacob. Anticipation gave way to disappointment over and over again as family members, nurses, hospital staff, and doctors paraded through the room, checking my temp, giving me meds, and asking how I was doing, blah, blah, blah. I just wanted to hold my son.

My husband, Dariel, finally convinced one nurse to go rogue and covertly sneak Jacob into my room. Despite the IV still attached to his head, the nurse gently laid him in my arms. For the second time in my life, it felt as though I held my heart in my hands. It seemed like an eternity had passed since I had heard Jacob's first cry and caught a brief glimpse of his naked behind immediately after delivering him.

Time stood still as I memorized his perfect face and studied his tiny hands and feet. I saw glimpses of my dad in his features and fought back the tears as I wished my father had lived to meet his grandson. The past nine months of swollen ankles, nausea, and seemingly endless doctor appointments melted away. I gently kissed his head, carefully avoiding the IV, and whispered in his ear, "I praise you for I am fearfully and wonderfully made," quoting Psalm 139 as I thanked God for another son.

We headed home from the hospital a few days later and picked up my firstborn son, Riley, who had been staying with his grandparents. We contently began our life as a family of four. In the first week, Jacob became jaundiced and lost weight, but we got him back on track and settled into our new routine. Everything seemed normal.

But at the regular newborn checkups, Jacob's head always measured in the ninety-ninth percentile (which means it was really big, as you can see in the picture below).

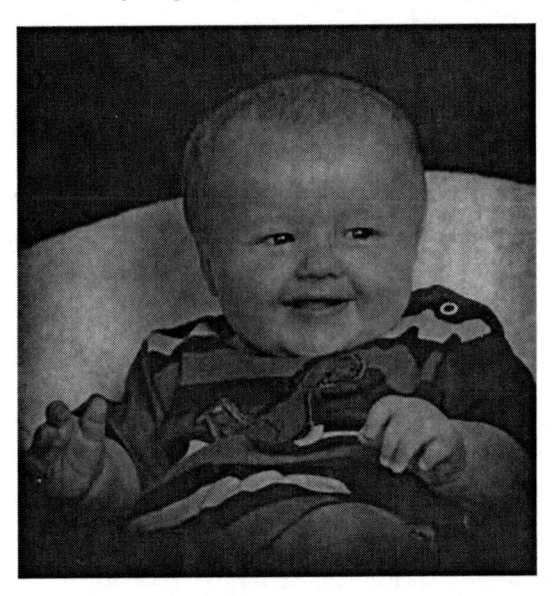

The pediatrician was concerned about possible brain issues, but an ultrasound when Jacob was six months old revealed there were no problems.

Despite the good report from the pediatrician, Dariel and I realized something seemed off and not quite normal. Jacob was exhibiting certain behaviors that had not been present in Riley nor would be present with our third son, Keaton, who came along two years after Jacob.

Early Development

Jacob never wanted a pacifier. If we gave him one, he would spit it out with such force that it sailed across the room. He rolled over, sat up, crawled, and began to walk much later than normal.

His potty-training also was very delayed. Even as late as four years old, we had to be diligent and consistent in monitoring his bathroom trips. To enroll in Pre-K3 at the private school Jacob attended, a child had to be potty-trained. Although Jacob turned three a full six months before preschool started, I held my breath every day waiting for the call that he had had an accident.

I consistently kept a change of underwear and pants in his school backpack, something I never had to do with his brothers who were potty-trained much more easily.

On the other hand, Jacob was verbal very early, speaking complete sentences at the age of one.

But he could not master the ability to sip through a straw despite repeated attempts and demonstrations—another skill that his older and younger brothers had no problem with.

One day, I went into the kitchen to prepare supper and seated Jacob on a blanket at one end of the kitchen so I could keep an eye on him as he played while I cooked. I placed a few of his favorite toys, a sippy cup filled with juice, and some crackers on the blanket to keep him occupied. After getting him settled, I turned the knob to preheat the oven and began digging in cabinets to find the dishes I needed. I was startled by a loud noise. Thinking that Riley had arrived to annoy his brother, I turned, expecting to begin to referee. To my surprise, the only person there was Jacob, who had thrown his sippy cup on the floor. I went over and handed it to him and had no more resumed my chef duties when he tossed it again. Before I could recover it one more time, he tossed one of his toys. I stood in amazement and watched as he threw another toy and then a cracker (which he promptly recovered and put in his mouth). Since he seemed more amused than upset, I returned to work in the kitchen and watched as he tirelessly threw anything he could reach on the floor. He then leaned or crawled to retrieve it and do it all over again. As this became a common source of self-entertainment, we finally figured out that Jacob was fascinated by the different sounds he created by throwing random items on the linoleum.

The Toddler Years

Jacob wore socks or went barefoot until he learned to walk. Dressing him for church, we proudly placed his first pair of shoes on his little feet. My husband and I looked at each other in horror as Jacob promptly sat on the floor, crying hysterically and refusing to move. He kept pointing at his shoes.

His first haircut? It broke my heart. No tantrum. Jacob just lowered his head while tears quietly flowed from his eyes.

There seemed to be some type of sensory issues too. My husband took Jacob to see his first movie, *Cats & Dogs*, when he was two-and-a-half years old. We weren't sure what to expect. Would the surround sound frighten him? Would he panic when the lights went down? The lights dimmed, and my husband whispered in Jacob's ear, "It's okay," as they waited patiently through the previews. Finally, the credits rolled and the action began. Dariel expected him to panic, but instead, Jacob rose to his feet, pointed his hand toward the screen, and excitedly announced to all who would hear, "I see cat! I see dog! I see movie!"

One thing was certain. Jacob didn't experience the world around him the way others did, but at this point, we didn't know if he was simply unique or truly had a problem. While these early developmental delays and peculiar behaviors caused some concern, the preschool years really began to raise some flags.

Preschool

I enrolled Jacob in a Mother's Day Out program at our church two days a week while I taught piano lessons. His classroom was downstairs; mine was upstairs. I had just started teaching my first student for the day when I heard loud screams coming from downstairs. I had a brief thought that someone wasn't happy in Mother's Day Out, but I continued teaching. Minute by minute, the screaming grew louder, inching closer to my room until the door swung open with such force that I jumped out of my chair. Jacob ran toward me, wailing at the top of his lungs, his arms flailing about and tears flowing. He threw himself on the floor in front of me, now bellowing and thrashing.

Embarrassed, I asked the teacher, Mrs. Black, what had happened. She stated she had no idea and seemed hesitant to admit that she didn't know what else to do. Several minutes of silent awkwardness prevailed until I told her I'd keep him with me until he calmed down and could return to class. Jacob's meltdown slowly subsided with me nearby, but I knew it wouldn't be the last time. In fact, it happened over and over again during his time in Mother's Day Out. There were days I couldn't handle even the thought of dealing with his meltdowns, so I just kept him with me.

We had experienced these meltdowns at home too, but we couldn't determine what triggered these episodes. Dariel and I just honestly didn't know what to do to stop them. Parenting tactics that had worked successfully with our other two children had zero effect with Jacob. If we sent him to his room for a time-out, he would completely shut down and stay in his room indefinitely without any verbal or physical expression. While most children ask to be removed from a time-out, Jacob would stay there until my husband or I told him the time-out was done. Our frustration and confusion grew as we struggled to help him.

When I began teaching music at our church's private school, we enrolled Jacob in the all-day Pre-K3 class. His class met for music on the first day of school, and I was his teacher. My child, who loved music and sang and danced at home with Mom, now stood in a corner and screamed during the entire class.

I made Jacob's lunch every day for preschool, a lunch that always included a peanut butter and jelly sandwich. The teacher informed me that he would not even attempt to eat the sandwich, which was cut in half, unless it was torn into small pieces.

Since I was teaching at the same school where Jacob was enrolled in Pre-K3 and then Pre-K4, I was constantly summoned to his classroom. He frequently experienced traumatic emotional meltdowns that seemed to last forever. Temper tantrums. Not the usual kind that come from not getting your way, but a tantrum born from sheer frustration. And when he was upset, he would shut down and refuse to even move.

I look back on the seemingly endless times I had to take Jacob into the nearest restroom at the school to calm him down or discipline him. I became frustrated when I couldn't get him to tell me what was wrong. I tried everything I knew. I scolded, pleaded, bribed, tried to make him laugh—nothing worked. I might as well have been doing a stand-up comedy routine in a room full of mannequins. No reaction, no verbal communication. Jacob simply froze for what seemed like hours. I was equal parts frustrated and afraid—frustrated that I, his mother, couldn't seem to reach him and afraid that there would come the day when I wouldn't be able to break through the wall of his shutdown at all.

Teachers were quick to offer their opinions. They commented that perhaps Jacob was a perfectionist, or maybe he didn't know how to obey, or any number of ideas to explain his behavior. I smiled and politely listened, wishing all the time that I could somehow disappear while the waves of embarrassment and shame washed over me. What must these people think of me as a parent? It was never-ending.

Kindergarten Woes

Then came kindergarten. Jacob's kindergarten teacher, Mrs. Sanders, invited me to observe Jacob's class one morning, and I looked on in horror as he rolled around the floor in constant movement during their daily routine. He wasn't making noise or being disrespectful; he just could not be still.

Mrs. Sanders' students received conduct marks each day of class based on colors. Green represented having the best behavior and red the worst. Much too often, when Mrs. Sanders saw me in the hall between classes or in the cafeteria, she'd head straight toward me to let me know how Jacob was doing that day. The majority of the time, it wasn't good. He was pretty consistent as a yellow, which fell between green and red.

The principal of the school, along with the kindergarten teacher, advised us to see a doctor so Jacob could be medicated for ADD (attention-deficit disorder). We grudgingly agreed to take him to the pediatrician, who was appalled that anyone would suggest giving Ritalin to a five-year-old child whether he had ADD or not.

Then came the almost weekly lectures from Mrs. Sanders, who admonished me to be strict with Jacob, to make him obey as she constantly shared stories about her strong-willed son who was now a wonderful young man. I just didn't have the strength anymore to defend myself or tell her we absolutely practiced obedience in our home. I nodded and smiled because I didn't know what to say.

Despite having the behavior issues in kindergarten, in Mrs. Sanders' class Jacob prayed to ask Jesus to be his savior and to receive Christ into his heart. My husband and I were obviously thrilled. We were also concerned about Jacob's understanding due to his young age, but we talked to him and asked him many questions over the next several weeks. We also arranged a meeting for Jacob to discuss his salvation with the children's pastor. A few months later, when we were sure Jacob was ready, he was baptized with all our family present. It was an amazing day despite the fact that the heater for the baptismal pool decided to stop working, and Jacob was immersed in extremely cold water. He handled it like a trooper and emerged from the water with a huge smile on his face.

Jacob didn't have any issues being immersed in the water for his baptism because we had a swimming pool in our backyard at home. He was very frightened and anxious when he first started getting in the pool, but Dariel and I worked with him, and in just a few weeks, he became very comfortable playing and splashing around with his brothers, even putting his head under the water.

Health Concerns

During Jacob's time in kindergarten, we went through a very disturbing experience. One day I was summoned to his classroom. He was sitting right outside the door and wouldn't move, complaining of extreme pain in his legs to the point that he couldn't walk. With assistance, I was able to get him into the van and to the emergency room of a local hospital. They rushed him into an exam room, took blood and urine samples, and ran a few other tests. After waiting for several hours, answering numerous questions, and talking to every nurse and doctor on duty, it seemed, we were told they could find nothing wrong. Since the pain had subsided by that time, the doctor told us to take him home and follow up with his pediatrician. Later that evening, Jacob remarked that it hadn't been a good day at all because "I had to give blood and pee in a cup." Yeah, that pretty much summed it up.

We were just a few hours into school the following day when I was summoned once again. This time Jacob was on the floor screaming in agony and complaining of severe leg pain. After getting him in the van, I rushed him to the pediatrician. A doctor and two nurses met me at the van and physically carried Jacob into the building as he writhed in agony and screamed even louder. At this point, I was a basket case, and my anxiety only grew as the doctor seemed helpless to understand what was going on.

The pediatrician's office called for an ambulance, and Jacob was loaded on the stretcher and placed into the ambulance as I climbed aboard and joined him for the bouncy, rocky drive to Texas Children's Hospital in the Texas Medical Center in Houston. The ride seemed to calm him down, and he was able to sleep during the time it took to transport him.

As they wheeled him through the emergency room doors and into the nearest exam room, Jacob woke up and once again began to complain of leg pain, but he seemed a little calmer than before. I experienced déjà vu as the door to the small exam room opened and closed repeatedly with a never-ending stream of doctors and nurses poking and prodding on my precious little boy.

I bounced between the phone on the wall (no cell phones allowed) and Jacob's bedside trying to update my husband, church family, and friends and attend to Jacob. Here we were for a second night in a different hospital waiting way too many hours. Finally, a doctor appeared, looked at me, and declared, "I'd like to try something." No explanation. Just that statement. At this point, I was willing to try anything, so I nodded my approval in a growing state of exhaustion, confusion, and fear.

Jacob sat up, drank a small cup of medicine, and the doctor disappeared.

Within ten minutes, I thought I'd finally gone over the edge and was having hallucinations.

My anxious son who had been riddled for hours with pain was suddenly "normal"—talking, laughing, playing—as if the last several agonizing hours were a distant memory.

What was happening?

Like a glorious vision, the doctor returned to check on Jacob. He was barely through the door when I asked, "What did you do?"

"I gave him medicine for anxiety," he explained. "I finally realized there was nothing physically wrong that we could determine, but he had somehow worked himself into a state of severe anxiety. So simply removing the anxiety would make it possible for him to return to normal."

"Then why was he screaming about the pain in his legs?" I asked.

"We think there was some type of pain in his legs, perhaps just growing pains. And for whatever reason, Jacob overreacted, and anxiety elevated what he was experiencing."

I accepted the doctor's explanation since Jacob's demeanor and behavior were living proof it had worked.

We wearily made the trip home and never had that problem with Jacob again. After the Asperger's syndrome diagnosis a year later and learning its symptoms, I had a better understanding of how this could happen (more on that later), but at the time, it was just one more thing to add to our growing list of "what is going on?"

Jacob also had a very unusual reaction to chronic ear infections. Through five years of age, he had numerous ear infections, which caused his eardrum to burst on five separate occasions. The first time it happened, we were all together in the playroom enjoying some family time when a dark liquid-like substance began oozing out of Jacob's ear. Dariel and I rushed him to the pediatrician. The minute the doctor walked into the exam room and saw Jacob's ear, he knew it was an ear infection because the goo coming out of Jacob's ear was the result of a burst eardrum. The pediatrician remarked that he didn't understand why Jacob hadn't complained of pain prior to the eardrum bursting because the time immediately before the eardrum eruption is excruciatingly painful. Unlike other children who would cry, complain, and tug on an ear with the pain of the ear infection, Jacob had remained silent.

When he was nine months old, Jacob had tubes placed in his ears to alleviate the persistent ear infections. At first, the tubes greatly reduced the number of ear infections, but as Jacob grew and the tubes began to move and eventually fall out altogether, the infections increased. When Jacob was five, I took him for a checkup at the ear, nose, and throat doctor because he had experienced another eardrum eruption. Jacob's hearing was tested, and remarkably, there was no hearing loss, but the doctor informed me that Jacob would have to have tubes placed in his ears again if there was another infection. Much to our amazement, the ear infections stopped, and Jacob's eardrum remained intact and healthy.

Denial

School was not the only venue where Jacob had issues. I was the pianist for the worship team and involved in rehearsals and church service performances on Sunday mornings from 8 a.m. until church was over, so my husband was the parent who was summoned when problems with Jacob arose, which was quite frequent. Dariel witnessed the same behavior I had to deal with during the school day. There were numerous meltdowns and shutdowns. The sweet Sunday school teachers had never seen anything like it, so my husband was pulled away from his technical duties in the sanctuary on a recurring basis.

The almost daily drama with Jacob was taking its toll. Were we inadequate parents? Why were we failing so miserably? I could see without a doubt a tremendous desire in Jacob to please others and that he had a tender, loving heart. Where was all this coming from?

I'm ashamed to admit it, but more often than not, I simply stuck my head in the sand and pretended there was nothing wrong. If I convinced myself everything was perfect, then it would be. Right? Sometimes I walked through the cafeteria during Jacob's lunch time at the private school and saw him sitting at the big, round table with his friends talking and laughing. He looked normal, didn't he? This could not be the same kid who had a meltdown two hours ago.

And then it happened. First grade began, and within two weeks, my precious six-year-old boy was asked to permanently leave Community Christian Academy. They no longer knew how to handle him. No more pretending that everything was fine. It wasn't. Would it ever be again? Where do we go from here?

2
AFTER THE DIAGNOSIS

But he said to me, "My grace is sufficient for you, for my power is made perfect in weakness."

—2 Corinthians 12:9

Expulsion

"I'm sorry, Mrs. Berry. We're going to have to ask Jacob to leave the school. We just don't know what to do with him."

Those were words I never wanted to hear and words I never expected to hear. I tried to pretend I was fine when the school principal broke the news, but the floor had just given way beneath me. I felt as if I were falling into a never-ending black hole.

The room was spinning. Anger. So much anger. Why couldn't the teacher just try? That witch! How could she do this to me? I mean, how could she do this to Jacob? Denial. Disbelief. They all converged on me at once. What could I say? How could I argue? I had seen it for myself, the seemingly never-ending requests to pull him from the classroom when his teacher didn't know what to do, the rolling on the floor in kindergarten, the meltdowns that couldn't be contained, and the shutdowns when he refused to move.

The expulsion came after Jacob walked into his first-grade class and noticed a folder attached to the dry eraser board with instructions for the day. He promptly flung himself on the floor into a screaming, crying mess.

When I finally got him calm enough to explain to me what happened, he told me he didn't understand what to do and got upset.

But that was it for the teacher. She was done and refused to even try. She wanted him out of her classroom, which led to his expulsion from the school.

And because the day couldn't get any worse, the principal, who had just informed us that Jacob had to leave the school, leaned down, got eye level with Jacob, shook his finger in his face and said, "And you, young man! Maybe one day you'll learn to obey."

I was infuriated. As a mom, an educator, or anyone, you don't speak to children that way, especially to a six-year-old who really had no understanding of what was happening.

I drove home in a daze, but I put on a happy face for Jacob. He was upset about having to leave school, not fully understanding. But I couldn't talk to him. Not yet. The pain and shame were still raw. If I admitted to him the whole truth about being expelled, I'd have to admit it to myself, too, and I wasn't ready. I comforted him as best I could.

The day got even darker when I had to deliver what I knew would be devastating news to Riley.

Meet the Family

From a young age, Riley was fiercely independent and mature. He never wanted to be singled out or have attention drawn to him in any way. He was a straight-arrow rule-follower throughout his school years. As parents, we loved that because we would never have to worry about Riley staying out too late, skipping school, or being willfully disobedient. Though not a perfect child, he definitely made his parents' lives easy.

Our youngest son, Keaton, was born after Jacob. After Keaton was born, my husband brought Jacob and Riley into the hospital room so they could meet their new brother. After getting Jacob and Riley to sit down, Dariel gingerly laid Keaton into Riley's arms. As soon as Dariel stepped back, Jacob whacked Keaton on the head with the small Thomas the Train toy he was holding. We scolded Jacob, even though it didn't seem to faze Keaton at all. Looking back, we consider it another one of Jacob's attempts to discover a new sound. He was curious to hear the sound produced when bouncing the toy train off his baby brother's head.

As soon as Keaton was mobile, he followed his big brothers around, wanting to do everything they did. All three of them slept in the same bedroom until Jacob was sixteen years old, even though our home had a bedroom for each of them. They kept their individual toys, clothes, and other things in their separate bedrooms, but at night they slept in the same room, with Riley and Keaton on bunk beds and Jacob on a twin bed.

Occasionally, my husband and I left our boys with my sister and her husband while we enjoyed a night out or had to be away for some other reason. Their aunt and uncle told us that when they were babysitting our boys, they witnessed Riley and Keaton being extremely protective of Jacob. As parents, we didn't see that in our

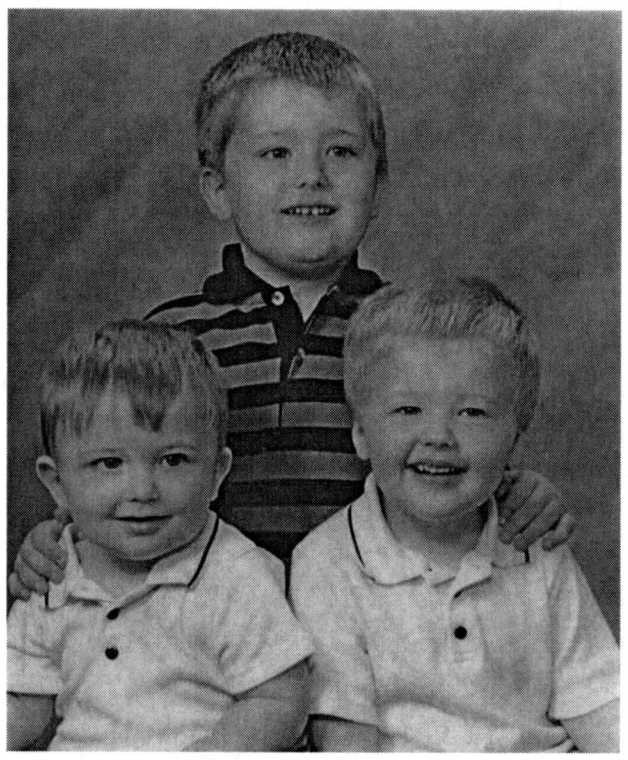

Back: Riley, age 4; Front from left: Keaton, age 16 months; Jacob, age 2

home very often, but the knowledge thrilled us and made us even more proud of our sons.

I was often asked by strangers if my sons were triplets when I had all three of them out in public. That question always made me laugh since there were two years between each of their births. Now, looking back at pictures of them, I can see the striking resemblance.

Riley, Jacob, and Keaton all attended the private school until Jacob's expulsion, riding to and from school each day together. But that time had now ended, and none of us were prepared.

Change Is Never Easy

I had to quit my job as the music teacher at the private school where the boys attended because I knew Jacob needed my attention. Without my job, there was no tuition discount, and we simply couldn't afford the school for Riley. I sat Riley down and explained as best I could to an eight-year-old that he would have to leave the only school he had ever known because we could no longer pay the tuition. Riley became angry and began to cry.

"Why does Jacob have to mess up? Why can't he stay at Eagle Heights? Why do I have to leave? Keaton doesn't have to leave!"

"No," I said. "Keaton is in Pre-K4 and is too young to attend public school. Your dad and I can afford to keep him there until he's old enough to go to public school."

"That's not fair! Why can't I stay? Why do I have to go too?" Riley demanded as his eyes began to fill with tears.

Then I remembered a scene from two years earlier. Dariel and I didn't have the money to pay for Riley's first grade tuition that year, so we put him in the local elementary public school. The second day of class, I drove past the school during his recess time to check on him. He was sitting in a corner of the playground all alone while his classmates flew high in the air on the swings, climbed on the jungle gym, and chased each other around in a game of tag. With a phone call to my mom who agreed to cover the tuition, we pulled Riley out the next day and put him back in Community Christian Academy.

Would it happen again with this new school? Would Riley make friends? Guilt poured over me, but I knew what had to be done.

Once more, I explained the day's events and how this would impact all of us. But all Riley could focus on was the huge change in his life, and he didn't want it. The sum total of everything that had occurred that horrible day came crashing in at once, and I lost it.

"Do you think I want to leave the school?" I shouted at him. "Do you think I want to give up my job? This isn't about you!"

No, at that precise second, much to my shame and reluctance to admit it, it was about *me*.

I had a bad day. *My* perfect routine life had been smashed to pieces by one despicable teacher and her cohort in crime, the school principal. *My* child wasn't perfect anymore. *I* was going to have to step out of my own bubble and try to figure out how to help my child with a problem that, as far as I knew, had no explanation.

I wanted it all to go away. I wanted yesterday when life was simple, when I had a great job that I loved and when all my kids were happily ensconced at their private school. I did not want to deal with any of this.

Sanity prevailed. The tears fell as I apologized to Riley, pulled him in for a hug, and held him tightly. Then I uttered the one, absolute truth that I hadn't been able to bring myself to say to him. "Riley, it is true that without the discount my teaching brings, we can't afford Community Christian. But," I paused and I struggled. "But I need you to walk into the new school every day with your brother. I don't think Jacob can do this without knowing you're there with him."

It was a lot to put on an eight-year-old, but it was the absolute truth. I didn't know yet what was going on, but I knew that Jacob needed help, and that help was going to have to come from everyone in our family.

The next day, I gathered myself together and took Riley and Jacob to the public elementary school we were zoned for. I talked to the principal and explained what had happened with Jacob at the private school.

With a total sense of dread, shame, and fear combining to make me an emotional mess, I watched as my two oldest sons were led from the school office to their new classrooms. They made it through the day, but Riley was not happy, and Jacob was still reeling from the change.

Acceptance

During that first day at Whispering Pines Elementary School, the school diagnostician tested Jacob and then delivered the news to Dariel and me. "Asperger's syndrome. Jacob has Asperger's syndrome."

What the heck is that? I didn't say it out loud.

The diagnostician answered my unspoken question by going into a lengthy description of Asperger's syndrome, but I didn't hear one word she said, or maybe I should say I didn't comprehend one word she said. To my ears, she sounded like the teacher in a Charlie Brown cartoon—"wah, wah, wah, wah," on and on. I just wanted to get out of there.

My husband and I practically crawled to our car. We didn't speak. We just stared straight ahead and tried to absorb what we had just been told.

As soon as we got home, I started researching online.

As I read the definition and symptoms of Asperger's syndrome, I told myself, *That doesn't sound at all like Jacob. They're crazy.*

A child with Asperger's syndrome doesn't make friends easily.

Jacob has friends.

A child with Asperger's syndrome may develop rituals such as getting dressed in a specific order.

Jacob doesn't do that.

A child with Asperger's syndrome may develop an intense, almost obsessive interest in a few areas, such as sports schedules, weather, or maps.

Jacob could care less about sports, weather, or maps.

Thank God for my husband. He read through everything, too, and said, "That sounds exactly like Jacob."

So I went back and looked at it again.

Children with Asperger's syndrome generally have difficulty interacting with others and are often awkward in social situations.

Yep.

A child with Asperger's syndrome may develop odd, repetitive movements such as hand wringing or finger twisting.

Well, there's that and saying the word pickle *over and over again.*

People with Asperger's syndrome tend to have problems understanding language in context and are very literal in their use of language.

Nailed it.

The movements of children with Asperger's syndrome may seem clumsy or awkward.

Ouch!

My husband was right. Every one of those absolutely described my son. I just couldn't admit it. There could not be anything wrong with my child. That made me a failure, right? Had I ingested something when I was pregnant that hurt him in the womb? I learned there was a possibility it could be hereditary. Okay, if that's true, then it must have come from my side of the family. More guilt.

I wallowed in all of it. *Why me? Why us? Why him? Why my family? I don't have time to deal with this.* Yes, pity and selfishness are not an attractive combination.

The Psychiatrist Speaks

My husband and I decided we wanted a second opinion. A good friend of ours had a son with Asperger's syndrome, and she recommended a psychiatrist. We made the appointment and soon had the confirmation. Yes, it was definitely Asperger's syndrome. The good news, if you can consider anything good at this point, was that it was a mild case.

As Dariel and I sat at the doctor's desk, her office door was ajar, and we all observed Jacob across the hall in a children's waiting room stocked with several toys. There was another child with his parent in the room with Jacob. We were fascinated to watch Jacob interact with the child. He was happy and friendly and talking. The doctor pointed out that Jacob's behavior at that moment was proof that his Asperger's syndrome was not an extreme case since typically a severe case would cause a child to avoid eye contact and certainly not desire to play with another child.

We asked the psychiatrist what the future held for Jacob as he became an adult. She told us that Asperger's syndrome, if left untreated, can cause obsessive-compulsive disorder or schizophrenia in adulthood. Not what you want to hear when you pretty much had his life mapped out before he was born. School, college, marriage, children, great job—now you're facing expulsion from school at six years old, a disorder you've never heard of, and the possibility of schizophrenia.

Your head spins. Your perfect world is rocked to the core, and you fall to your knees seeking direction and comfort from the only One who can make sense of it all.

Since the doctor mentioned obsessive-compulsive disorder, we informed her that for several weeks Jacob had been randomly saying the word *pickle*. Despite not knowing at the time he had Asperger's syndrome, we were somewhat concerned about his inability to control himself. She said that was typical. Asperger's syndrome causes people to make repetitive gestures or shout out random words like Jacob was doing.

We asked the doctor how to stop the behavior, fearing the worst. Perhaps they would have to administer electric shock to Jacob or submit him to some other horrible treatment. Time froze for a moment as we inwardly cringed and waited for some awful remedy.

"You just tell him to stop," the doctor said.

Awkward pause. We waited for the other shoe to drop. She just smiled.

"Seriously?" I said. "That's it?"

"Yes."

It's called parenting. Simple as that. We put the kibosh on the word *pickle* immediately.

Jacob didn't stop saying it overnight, but within a week, the pickle was shown the door. Sometime later, Jacob began making an odd, circular gesture with his right hand. Again, this compulsion happened at random times. It took several days for my husband and me to realize this too had to go the way of the pickle. Every time we observed him making the gesture, we told him to stop. It, too, took only a few days to disappear forever.

Who knew? It's funny now to think how certain Dariel and I were that we were going to have to climb some difficult mountain when it only took diligent parenting to correct the problem.

After successfully conquering those two compulsions, there hasn't been a new one in twelve years. As Jacob got older, we explained to him how people with Asperger's syndrome have the tendency to develop obsessive-compulsive disorder. We wanted to make him aware and hopefully prevent any other issues.

The psychiatrist also wrote us an official letter detailing Jacob's diagnosis and included aspects of this fairly new disorder known as Asperger's syndrome.

> To Whom It May Concern:
>
> Jacob Berry is a patient under my psychiatric care. Jacob has been diagnosed with Asperger's syndrome. It is my understanding that he continues to have difficulties with behavior in the school setting, particularly in the area of physical education. I hope that I can be helpful in articulating how to best help Jacob when he becomes overwhelmed and then proceeds to "shut down," which may appear as oppositional behavior to outside observers. The following is an excerpt from *Handbook of Autism and Pervasive Developmental Disorders* by Fred Volkmar et al. This section is devoted to behavioral management of individuals with Asperger's syndrome.
>
> Challenging behaviors are common among individuals with AS. As noted, their motivations are rarely malicious and are more likely to stem from difficulties with arousal regulation and poor emotional insight into self and others.

Specific problem-solving strategies, usually following a verbal algorithm, may be taught for handling the requirements of frequently occurring, troublesome situations (involving novelty, intense social demands, or frustration). Training is usually necessary for recognizing situations as troublesome and for selecting the best available learned strategy to use in such situations. Cognitive and behavioral strategies for anxiety management (e.g., breathing exercises) are often helpful in teaching students to control negative emotion. In designing any intervention to control problematic behaviors, it is important to collect data to both understand the function that they are serving to the child (i.e., using functional behavioral analysis) and to ascertain a true estimate of the efficacy of treatment.

In thinking about Jacob and how to succeed in school, please consider the above. My belief is that new situations that are unfamiliar to him very easily overwhelm him. When he is overwhelmed, he needs a specific, consistent way to help him. Initially, he may need more direct direction to get him over the challenge of the new situation. In time, coming up with a problem-solving algorithm may be helpful as well. I have suggested to his parents the idea of practicing the activities in physical education class prior to actually having to do it so that the activity is not novel to him. Hopefully, this will help solve the problem. If this does not, it is important to understand that this is not simply oppositional behavior. In addition, I still support the notion of adaptive physical education for this young man. Motor skills in children with Asperger's syndrome are not as adept as other children, which may explain his continued struggles with this area. By adaptations in this area, we would be able to "level the playing field" for him to be successful.

It was with great delight that I returned to the private school from which Jacob had been expelled, with that letter firmly gripped in my hand. I first located the principal who had shook his finger in Jacob's face and admonished my son to learn how to obey. I gleefully handed a copy of the doctor's letter to him and informed him that a child with Asperger's syndrome may possess an inability to follow certain instructions and directives, an effect that in no way can be defined as disobedience but rather a symptom of the disorder. This symptom causes extreme fear and anxiety, which in turn produces the noncompliant behavior. While I was on a roll, I made my way to Jacob's kindergarten teacher and relayed to her the same information. I let both the principal and the teacher know that I sincerely hoped that they would learn from this experience that children are not all made the same and cannot always be judged by the same standard.

Once Jacob started attending Whispering Pines Elementary, we participated in Jacob's first ARD (admission, review, and dismissal) meeting. An ARD meeting is required for all children being placed in the special education program. Jacob was put on an individual education plan (IEP), and my husband and I were given a booklet called *Procedural Safeguards*. The purpose of the book is to inform parents, as well as the child, of the rights and protections they have according to the law.

Jacob was officially diagnosed and classified as a special education student with a condition listed on the autism spectrum.

What in the world do we do now? Where do we go from here?

The self-pity and self-loathing had mercifully disappeared, and now there only remained a fierce determination. We were going to kick this in the butt. And we were just getting started.

3
HELP WANTED

Likewise the Spirit helps us in our weakness. For we do not know what to pray for as we ought. And we know that for those who love God all things work together for good, for those who are called according to his purpose.
—Romans 8:26, 28

The Road to Discovery
Asperger's syndrome is a type of pervasive developmental disorder (PDD) characterized by difficulties in nonverbal communication and social interaction, obsessive and repetitive patterns of behavior and interests, as well as physical clumsiness and atypical language. Although

Asperger's syndrome is on the autism spectrum, children with Asperger's syndrome typically function better than those with autism. Asperger's syndrome was named after Austrian pediatrician Hans Asperger, who first described the disorder in 1944. However, Asperger's syndrome was not standardized as a diagnosis until the 1990s.

Jacob was born in 1999 and diagnosed in 2005. Asperger's syndrome was still new, and as we inquired and researched, no one really knew the best way to help him. The psychiatrist told us that behavior modification was the key.

Before we found the psychiatrist who confirmed Jacob's diagnosis, Dariel and I desperately began to seek help for Jacob, devouring information on what we could do to work with him.

First, we took him to a Christian counselor who very humbly and wisely informed us that Jacob's issues were not included in the scope of her training. She assured us that he was an emotionally happy and well-adjusted little boy and that we were doing a great job of parenting. Wonderful news, except we still had no clue what was going on with our own child. And while hearing "you are great parents" is amazing, we still felt like failures.

Not giving up, we found a psychologist. Jacob charmed the psychologist with his witty banter and funny stories. At the end of the session, she told me that Jacob was great one on one, but he needed a group of his peers to interact with.

"Where do I find that?" I asked.

"I have no idea," she said.

Questions Asked and Answered

After weekly sessions with the specialist at school and seeing a counselor, a psychologist, and then a psychiatrist, Jacob knew something was up. He was young, but he had questions. I was in the bedroom putting away a load of laundry one night when I looked up and saw Jacob walking toward me.

"Mom, why have I been going to see all these doctors? What's going on?"

I sat down on the bed for a minute. We were several months into this journey, and we hadn't told him anything. We didn't know how. We were still wrapping our heads around it ourselves.

I took a deep breath. "Jacob, remember when you had to leave school a few months ago?" He nodded. "Well, we knew there was something going on with you, so we've been taking you to different doctors trying to figure out exactly what it is and how we can help you." My voice cracked as I attempted to hold my emotions in check. "Jacob, you have something called Asperger's syndrome. Your dad and I aren't exactly sure what all that means, but here is one thing I do know. This is going to be difficult. Really hard. But we're going to do this together, and one day you're going to come out on the other side of this with an amazing testimony. God is going to use you to help others."

Jacob nodded and said, "Okay." Then he proceeded back to his room. He had an explanation, and at the moment, that was all he needed to hear.

I knew what I had told him wasn't a lie, an exaggeration, or a Pollyanna promise to make him feel better. It was the truth, and I knew it was the truth the moment the words left my mouth. Looking back, I am certain that it was the Holy Spirit speaking hope, comfort, and wisdom into Jacob's young heart and also into mine.

But what now? I had to get Jacob started on the road to meet this syndrome head on.

While seeking God's direction in prayer, I began reading, researching, and making phone calls.

I finally located a group that had behavior modification classes in Jacob's age group. The only problem was that it required a 45-minute drive one way in good traffic. I met with them, liked what I heard, and registered Jacob for the class. I wasn't sure how I was going to get him there once a week and make the drive since I also had to care for Riley and Keaton, but I was determined. I'd get it done because Jacob had to be there.

One week before Jacob was to begin the class, a friend showed me a local newspaper article about a woman who had a business called Behavior Plus. In the article, she mentioned Asperger's syndrome. I immediately called and peppered her with questions. She was located only five minutes from our home. I figured I'd give it a shot at least for a few months, and if it didn't work, we'd try the facility that was 45 minutes away.

The actual journey, our way back, our true beginning started here—with Nancy Kling and Behavior Plus.

Receiving Jacob's diagnosis had sent me falling into what seemed an unending pit of fear, despair, and uncertainty. I had spent the last several months desperately trying to claw and fight myself out from the darkness and confusion. Finally, this horrific time in our lives began to see a light of hope, of answered prayer, of a future.

4
FIRST STEPS

Be strong and courageous. Do not be frightened, and do not be dismayed, for the Lord your God is with you wherever you go.

—Joshua 1:9

Overcoming the Guilt

Jacob attended the weekly behavior group at Behavior Plus with Mrs. Kling as the coach. Parents were required to attend the last twenty minutes of the hour-long session to observe and learn what had taken place. Honestly, in the beginning it was so difficult for me to watch Jacob's group in those final twenty minutes that I often asked my husband to do it.

I had a preconceived idea of how my beloved child interacted with other children at school, at birthday parties, in Sunday school, and so on. Being held prisoner in a small room to observe that same beloved child attempting to socialize with other kids his age was painful. He had strange gestures and movements, and he blurted out statements that were at times random or inappropriate for the moment. Often the kids played a game, and I had to stop myself numerous times (parents weren't allowed to speak, only observe) from correcting Jacob's behavior. He interrupted the coach, made noises, and offered weird comments. It was so awkward that I cringed and had to look away.

The first few times I attended the parental observation time, the enormity of what we were dealing with hit me. I couldn't stop thinking, as a teacher myself, how difficult it must have been for Jacob's teachers, and I was finally able to let go of the misplaced anger at the private school teacher who was the catalyst for Jacob's expulsion.

I struggled with the memories of taking Jacob from his Pre-K3 or Pre-K4 class and into the bathroom to discipline him because the teacher had asked me to come down and deal with his latest shutdown or meltdown. Waves of guilt poured over me as I realized that I too had assumed Jacob had behavior issues.

The more I learned and observed, the more I was able to finally begin forgiving myself as I realized the expulsion, Jacob's meltdowns, and his seemingly eccentric behavior at times were not the result of my failure as a parent. Asperger's syndrome is what it is. It was not going away, and my husband and I had much work to do.

Beginning to Understand

A few weeks after Jacob was diagnosed, he attended physical and occupational therapy as prescribed by the psychiatrist. The doctor had informed us that Asperger's syndrome causes changes in the senses and can affect coordination. Although I had Riley and Keaton with me, I was able to observe the therapist working with him a few times. I was shocked that Jacob couldn't complete basic tasks. He wasn't able to climb during one exercise. He failed to work his way out of a tub filled with balls. He couldn't catch a plastic ball tossed to him that should have been easy to catch.

It was so difficult to watch him struggle, but I was beginning to understand many things—the delayed start in his crawling and walking, his inability to sip through a straw, his fascination with dropping items on the kitchen floor because of the difference in his sense of sound, his peculiar response to leg pain and ear infections, and his extreme reaction to wearing shoes the first time. I even learned later that his large head was also a sign of Asperger's syndrome.

When I asked the occupational therapist about Jacob's inability to sit still in Mrs. Sanders' kindergarten class, she explained to me that in group settings where other children are comfortable sitting on the floor, Asperger's syndrome kids often sit in a chair or even on a large, bouncy ball. Their difficulty in remaining still and focused while sitting on the floor has to do with their sensory issues.

Little by little, memory by memory, it was all beginning to make sense.

A Painful Start

Life at Whispering Pines Elementary School was not going well. Isn't that a charming school name? Doesn't it stir visions of beautiful trees in a country setting with ducks floating lazily on the adjacent pond? I wish. It had become my worst nightmare. Within its halls ensued a daily battle between my six-year-old Asperger's syndrome son, his teachers, and the administrators. Although we were meeting with the psychiatrist and attending a behavior group, Jacob was still having a really difficult time. Whispering Pines repeatedly called me to the school to bring Jacob out of his latest meltdown.

One particular day, my cell phone rang, interrupting my morning errands. I noticed the caller ID, and my stomach twisted into a large knot. *Not again*, I thought.

It was Jacob's school. Why did I think that I'd actually make it through one eight-hour school day without having to do this again? I wasn't sure I could do this again.

"Hello?" I should have said, "I know. I need to come up there." But there was the smallest glimmer of hope that this time it might be good news.

I was wrong. As usual.

"Yes. Okay. I'm on my way."

I pulled into my usual parking spot and sat for a few seconds, willing myself to walk in. I got out of the van and prayed with every step. *God, give me strength. God, give me wisdom. God, show me what do.*

I opened the front door of the school and stopped in my tracks, frozen with a combination of fear and despair. I could literally hear Jacob from somewhere deep within the bowels of the school as he screamed and cried.

I fought the urge to collapse into a sobbing, despondent, confused heap of a mess right there in the lobby. But I calmly walked into the office. I didn't have to tell them who I was or why I was there. Another day, another Jacob episode, and Mom to the rescue.

I was taken into the office of the principal, Mrs. Eastman.

"Mrs. Berry." *Julie, I thought. Surely we're on a first name basis by now.* I just nodded.

"I'm sorry to have to call you again today." *I'm sorry too. More sorry than you could possibly know.*

"Jacob has had another episode." *Shock, surprise, not.*

"We can't get him to move, so we're unable to bring him down here. He's just standing in the hall." *No, he's not just standing in the hall. He's screaming and crying AND standing in the hall.*

"No problem," I cheerfully pronounced as I died a little more inside.

They marched me down the hall. I felt like a death row inmate being led to execution.

The wailing grew louder as we approached. I wasn't sure how much more I could endure. It felt as if a giant, invisible hand had reached inside my chest to squeeze out my heart.

We turned the corner, and there he was.

He looked up at me with fear all over his face, tears flowing down his cheeks. His demeanor instantly changed when he saw me. Fight became hope. Fear began to subside. Mom was there.

But he didn't run to me or reach out to me or ask for help. The shutdown caused by Asperger's syndrome had a firm grip and wouldn't let go, not even when Mom appeared.

You would think at this point that I'd walk over and give him a big hug and tell him everything was all right. I wanted to, but I knew I couldn't. That doesn't work with Asperger's syndrome—not if you ever want to see your child overcome these moments.

Any outsider witnessing this whole event would have given me the worst-mom-of-the-year award, and I would have accepted it. But I had to use the methods we were learning. I had to be strong. I had to get him back in his classroom to finish his day, even though all I wanted to do was scoop him up, hold him tight, run away, and never look back.

"Jacob, can you tell me what's wrong?"

He looked at me as the tears continued to fall, but he wouldn't say a word.

"Jacob, talk to me. You and Dad and I have talked about this. You can't ignore us."

Silence. Tears.

"Jacob. Talk to me. It's okay. I just want to help you." More silence. A stoic teary-eyed face met mine. I waited. And waited. "Jacob, talk to me."

"I didn't understand," he finally spoke.

"What didn't you understand?"

He began to sob. "Mrs. Shaw said we needed to go sit in a group, but I didn't know which group."

How could I help him? How could I heal this hurt? How could I help him defeat this fear?

I looked at the principal. "Mrs. Eastman, can you let Mrs. Shaw know what happened?"

"Absolutely," she said.

I turned my attention to Jacob. "Is that okay, Jacob? Mrs. Shaw can show you where to go."

He hesitantly nodded his head.

"Are you okay to go back into class now?" I asked.

Again, he nodded, knowing that he needed to return to class but not sure he could.

"Jacob, I love you. I'll see you this afternoon, okay?"

"Love you, too," he answered quietly as he took Mrs. Eastman's hand. Together, they slipped inside the classroom away from my sight.

I quickly wound my way back through the seemingly endless maze of halls, walked out the front door, and collapsed behind the steering wheel of our van. I hadn't wanted anyone in the school to see me break down. I desperately needed everyone to think I was strong and in control. But I wasn't. Far from it. I cried as feelings of helplessness washed over me.

I needed to save Jacob just as I'd always needed to save those I loved. Growing up with an alcoholic mother had paved the wave for me to be a dutiful, helpful person who never wanted anyone to experience pain or sorrow. I couldn't save my mom, and despite my greatest wish, I knew I couldn't save Jacob either. I couldn't, and I wouldn't. Jacob had to learn to overcome his fears, and I had to hand over my fear to God and trust him as we walked through this together.

I wept, and a thousand selfish thoughts ran through my head. *Why is this happening to us? Why is this happening to Jacob? What do I do? Will he ever get better? Will I have to come to school every day from now until he graduates? I can't do it. I'm a terrible mother for thinking that. I'm a terrible mother because I'm helpless to help my child.*

With shaking hands, I dug into my purse to find my cell phone.

"Dariel," I said when my husband answered the phone, "I can't do this anymore."

"What?" he answered, trying to put my statement in some type of context.

"You're just going to have to take care of this. I can't handle it. It's killing me."

"What?" he patiently asked again.

"I had to come back to Whispering Pines again today."

"Jacob?"

"Yes. I—I can't take it."

"It will be okay. I will come if you need me to."

"No, I can do it." I pulled it together. "I know it's stupid to ask you to drive an hour from work to come here. I just don't know what to do."

"Neither do I," he admitted. "We'll get through this. We'll do whatever we have to for Jacob."

Slow and Steady

I can't begin to remember how many times this scenario occurred in the first few months. But as we continued the sessions at Behavior Plus, things began to improve. Jacob was finally settling into a routine. His first-grade teacher, Mrs. Shaw, was patient and willing to work with us to do whatever she could to help Jacob.

One of the first things we discovered was that change was a big struggle for Jacob. One day in first grade, he walked into the school cafeteria for lunch and headed to the spot where he normally sat. But the tables had been rearranged, and the confusion of where to sit simply overwhelmed him. He promptly turned around, walked out of the cafeteria, and began to cry. Initially shutdown and unable to talk, Jacob eventually told the teacher what had happened. This was a major improvement. I wasn't called to help him because he was able to stop the meltdown and communicate.

The principal relayed the cafeteria story to me and shared the fact that she had never encountered this reaction from a student in all her years in education.

Jacob's other big challenge was tackling any new activity. Although there was no issue with his physical education class in the private school, that class was exceptionally difficult at Whispering Pines Elementary. If the coach had to explain a new game, exercise, or drill, Jacob would totally shut down. So many directions being given at once, paired with the paralyzing fear that he wouldn't be able to do the activity correctly, overwhelmed him.

Another fact that we had learned from the psychiatrist was that the fear of being wrong, whether it is answering a question or attempting a new activity, could paralyze Asperger's syndrome kids. The doctor told us, for example, that if a teacher asked a question and the Asperger's syndrome child was 99 percent certain he knew the correct answer, he still would not raise his hand or attempt to answer because of the overwhelming fear of being wrong.

Effective Strategies

At home and school, we implemented several of the strategies we learned from Nancy Kling, Jacob's behavior coach. The principal and teachers gladly embraced any plan that would assist Jacob.

First was the Cup, a technique explained in the book *The Cup Kid* by Nancy Kling*. Since Jacob's shutdowns often impeded his ability to communicate verbally, Mrs. Shaw kept a picture of a cup on her desk with the numbers 1 through 5 written on it. If Jacob was having a difficult time, Mrs. Shaw had him point to a number on the cup. The number indicated the extent to which Jacob's cup was full. The higher the number, the fuller the cup. Arrangements had been made between the administration, teacher, and Mrs. Kling that if Jacob's cup was ever full or close to being full, he would be taken out of class to a safe environment where he could engage in an activity that would empty his cup. One such activity that helped him was drawing. The idea was to allow Jacob to empty the cup before it ran over. This strategy helped Jacob communicate anxiety before it blew up into a meltdown in front of his peers. It also developed trust with his teachers at the school.

We also used the strategy Expected and Unexpected Behaviors (www.socialthinking.com). When Jacob's lack of social skills caused him to speak or act in an inappropriate manner, instead of scolding him or punishing him, we asked him, "Jacob, was that expected or unexpected behavior?" His training in behavior modification was helping him understand what acceptable behaviors looked like. This simple exercise caused Jacob to stop and

---

*Nancy Kling, The Cup Kid: Parenting a Child with Meltdowns (Friendswood, TX: Come Along Publishing, 2008).

think about what had happened. Over time, that thought process occurred before he reacted, and eventually the unexpected behavior stopped altogether.

His teachers learned how to handle his shutdowns. If Jacob was unresponsive verbally, he was given the opportunity to write and draw what he was feeling. This technique became a tremendous asset in helping Jacob communicate what was causing a meltdown or shutdown.

He also began keeping a Behavior Notebook. He carried it with him at all times, and at the completion of each class, his teacher placed a check mark beside a desired behavior that had been accomplished. Jacob's father and I had to sign the notebook every night as part of his homework. We poured over the chart and praised the check marks he'd received. If there was a behavior that hadn't been checked off, we inquired what happened, discussed whether the behavior was expected or unexpected, and decided on a strategy for the next day.

This method also had a name—the Do Over. When Jacob explained that he didn't receive a check mark beside a desired behavior, we asked him, "What would you do over to receive the check mark if you could go back and do it again?" He came up with some ideas, or we helped him determine a desired behavior. Each time, it again reinforced the expected behavior.

One of Jacob's favorite tools learned at Behavior Plus was Superflex, a superhero social thinking curriculum created by Michelle Garcia Winner and Stephanie Madrigal (www.socialthinking.com). The Superflex curriculum provided fun, motivating ways to teach Jacob (and other children with Asperger's syndrome as well as other diagnosed social difficulty disorders) how to build his social abilities. It worked by teaching him that Superflex is the superhero ability inside him that helps him defeat his social challenges (represented as characters called Unthinkables) by using flexible thinking.

Jacob skirmished with many of the Unthinkables, but his primary battles were with two of the most notorious—Rock Brain and Glass Man.

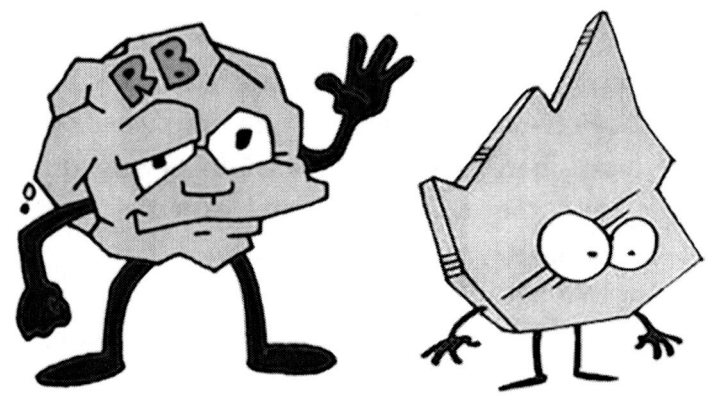

ROCK BRAIN GLASS MAN
Copyright © 2017 Think Social Publishing, Inc.
All Rights Reserved. www.socialthinking.com

Rock Brain is the Unthinkable we encouraged Jacob to defeat when a shutdown reared its ugly head. Rock Brain claimed victory on occasion, but Superflex Jacob learned to fight him off more frequently. Glass Man was the Unthinkable who caused those huge meltdowns that found Jacob crying, screaming, and throwing himself on the floor. Jacob fought many valiant battles against Glass Man and struck him down more and more often.

Several months into Jacob's first-grade year, the coaches at Behavior Plus began working with the staff of Whispering Pines on how to help Jacob. Prior to Jacob's admission to the school, they had never encountered a problem this severe.

I can't say enough how amazing this partnership was between the school and Behavior Plus. The tools Jacob was learning at Behavior Plus were being reinforced at home and at school. I truly believe this teamwork was instrumental in Jacob's remarkable improvement during his time at Whispering Pines Elementary School.

But—and there is always a *but*—we also had our issues. Things weren't all puppy dogs and roses. Before the teamwork, there were some major hurdles to overcome.

5
I WILL FIGHT YOU

Paul said to the centurion who was standing by, "Is it lawful for you to flog a man who is a Roman citizen and uncondemned? So those who were about to examine him withdrew from him immediately, and the tribune also was afraid, for he realized that Paul was a Roman citizen and that he had bound him.

—Acts 22:25, 29

I'm a Christian, but I'm also a mom. Just as the apostle Paul stood up for his rights as a Roman citizen in Acts 22, I didn't hesitate to fight for the rights of my son.

It was a Friday afternoon around 2:15 p.m. My cell phone rang. The caller ID showed it was Jacob's school.

"Mrs. Berry, we're going to have to expel Jacob from school for two days," the principal, Mrs. Eastman, informed me.

"What? Why? What did he do?" I exclaimed as I almost ran the car off the road.

"For indecent exposure."

"Are you kidding me?"

Without going into more detail, the principal asked me to come to the school, and that's exactly where I headed.

Two days earlier, I had purchased Jacob a new package of underwear, but I didn't wash them before he wore them. The next day, he had a rash, and his dad applied some topical medicine to the affected area.

The following day at school, Jacob's rash began to itch when he was at lunch. Since they were not allowed to go to the bathroom during lunch, he removed his pants just enough so he could scratch the inflamed area. Some of the students saw him, and within minutes he was taken by a teacher to the office for exposing himself.

When I arrived at the school, Mrs. Eastman met me immediately and told me what had happened. I explained to her about the underwear and the rash it had created.

"Well, Mrs. Berry, I'm sorry. There's nothing I can do."

"Seriously?" I exclaimed. "You know he has Asperger's syndrome and he's only six years old. He had no idea what he was doing. You *know* that."

Then I realized it was almost 3:00 p.m.—dismissal time for school each day—and that this had happened during Jacob's lunch time around 11:30 a.m.

"Where has Jacob been all this time?" I asked Mrs. Eastman. "If you brought him to your office before lunch was over, has he been in here this whole time?"

"Yes," she replied.

"Then why was I not called until after 2:00 p.m.?"

She stammered and stuttered and changed the subject, but I knew. I knew the reason. They waited to notify me as late as possible on a Friday so I wouldn't be able to take any action until Monday, and his expulsion was for Monday and Tuesday. But the principal had no idea who she was dealing with.

One more time, Mrs. Eastman stated, "I'm sorry. There's nothing I can do."

I looked her straight in the eye and said, "I will fight you."

Her reply? "Do what you have to do."

When we got home, I talked to Jacob. It broke my heart. He didn't understand the full scope of what had transpired. "Mom, it itched and I had to scratch it." He was six years old!

He had no clue that he had done anything wrong.

I was beyond furious. I was a woman—no, a mother—on a mission.

Online, I researched lawyers who specialized in children with special needs. I was coming up empty until I found a website for an Asperger's syndrome support group located in the Houston area. I called and spoke to a person who recommended a lawyer in Round Rock, Texas, outside of Austin. I contacted the law firm but didn't expect to reach anyone since we were already headed into the weekend. As I expected, my call went to voicemail where I left a detailed message.

Much to my surprise, my phone rang early Saturday morning. It was the lawyer from Round Rock. I told him what had happened, and he listened patiently. My blood began to boil again as I recounted the story.

Then he asked, "Mrs. Berry, what do you want to happen?"

I didn't even hesitate. "I want them to pay. I want to sue them for everything they've got. And it's not about money. It's about them not *ever* doing this again to my son."

I was angry and out for revenge, but fortunately, God sent me a lawyer who had ethics and a heart for parents dealing with these kinds of issues. He offered to send an advocate employed with his firm to our home to teach my husband and me our rights and what to do in cases like this. The lawyer and I agreed that we would use what we learned from the advocate and contact the school district on Monday. If I did not receive the response I desired from the district, we would proceed with legal action.

The advocate drove straight from Round Rock and arrived at our home around 8:00 p.m. Saturday evening. We spent two hours with him, asking questions, taking notes, and learning. The advocate brought literature that explained our rights as parents of a special needs child. We were informed, sadly, that schools typically offer the minimum services available to children of special needs in an attempt to save money. He also made us aware of our rights under the Americans with Disabilities Act (ADA), for which Jacob qualified.

What we found the most amazing, and also the most disturbing, was when the advocate abruptly held up a copy of the *Procedural Safeguards* we had received during the ARD meeting and placed it against his forehead, facing out. He asked us to look at the booklet and tell him what year was printed on the cover. My husband and I both responded, "2001."

He put the book down on the table, looked at us, and waited. It took a few minutes to sink in, but suddenly we saw the light.

"It's 2006!" I shouted.

"Exactly. The school didn't even provide you with an up-to-date copy."

The advocate patiently taught us about our rights and the school district's requirements. After a two-hour session and seemingly endless questions, he gathered up his things and proclaimed that we were ready. We thanked him profusely as we walked him to his car.

Alone once again, Dariel and I marveled at God's provision and headed for bed, mentally exhausted but prepared to go into battle.

When Monday morning arrived, I was on my phone with the school at 7:20 a.m. I knew what to ask for, what to say, and what buttons to push. I asked to see Jacob's entire file, which included everything since he was enrolled. It included all the initial testing and forms that had been set up during his ARD meeting.

The school directed me to the school district's Special Education Department. I walked into the office with Jacob in tow, approached the receptionist, and asked to see all of Jacob's records.

After she handed the file to me, I took everything to my car and searched through all the pages. Much to my shock, there was no Behavior Intervention Plan (called a BIP for short). I shuffled through all the papers two more times just to make sure, but the BIP was nowhere to be found.

I walked back into the office, shoved the file at the receptionist, and said, "Show me Jacob's BIP."

She rifled through the papers for a minute and then said, "Let me go get Dr. Richards. I'll be right back."

Jacob and I took a seat in the lobby and waited and waited. And we waited some more. I was laughing on the inside. I had them. I knew it.

Eventually, the head of the department, Dr. Richards, came to get me. He escorted Jacob and me to his office. "Mrs. Berry, we seem to have a problem."

You think?

"We can't, uh, seem to find a BIP for Jacob."

"Well, that's a big problem," I replied. "Due to some of the behavioral issues he's been having at Whispering Pines, a Behavior Intervention Plan is required, and the school did not provide one for Jacob. They had no problem expelling him, a child diagnosed with Asperger's syndrome and classified special ed. I spent two hours with an advocate this weekend, and I know for a fact that the school is negligent for not providing a BIP for Jacob."

Jacob was occupying himself by playing with toys, oblivious to what was going on, but I wanted to jump up and down and do cartwheels.

Dr. Richards rambled on for a few minutes about how I was absolutely right and they would correct it as soon as possible. He tried his best to be super friendly and helpful, smelling a lawsuit on the horizon.

I interrupted his endless excuses and promises and said, "I want Jacob back in school *now*, and I want this expulsion *completely* removed from his record."

"Of course, of course. I'll call the principal right now and get Jacob back in class."

Score!

I took Jacob by the hand and calmly walked down the hall and out the front door. I unlocked the van, got Jacob settled in his car seat, scooted behind the steering wheel, and placed the key in the ignition.

"Yes!" I fist-bumped the air. "Yes!"

The victory was sweet, but I was still not happy that this had happened to my sweet, innocent little boy.

Anxiously, I awaited Dr. Richards' call to let me know he had cleared things up with the principal so Jacob could return to school. A couple of hours later, the call came, but the news was not anything I wanted to hear.

"I've called Mrs. Eastman twice," he said, "and she won't take my calls. I'm driving over to the school now to talk to her in person."

"Thank you," I muttered, and hung up the phone.

"You have got to be kidding!" I yelled out loud. "She is doing this on purpose because I told her I would fight her. I won, and now she doesn't want to face the truth."

I called my husband who, as usual, was the voice of calm and sanity. He wisely told me just to wait. It took everything in me not to hop in the car, drive to that school, and let the principal have it with both barrels. I prayed for patience and understanding, but I'll admit that I wanted her to hurt like Jacob and my family had hurt when she booted him out of school.

Deep breaths. More prayer. I could do this.

The phone rang again about thirty minutes later, and Dr. Richards told me Jacob could return to school. I wanted to ask him what Mrs. Eastman had said when she heard the news, but I held my tongue. It was time to put it behind me and get back to helping Jacob succeed.

I had told the principal I would fight. I did, and I won. He was back in school.

We Have an Advocate

There were a few more battles on our journey. Several months later, desiring the absolute best for Jacob after the indecent exposure incident, Dariel and I hired a local advocate to attend Jacob's second ARD meeting with us. His fee was quite high, but when it was over, it was well worth every penny.

When the meeting started, our advocate jumped right in and asked all the school employees sitting around the large conference table to state their names, positions at the school, and any training they had received in working with Asperger's syndrome students.

You could have heard a pin drop. The color drained from most of their faces.

Each school official then answered the advocate's questions, but not one of them could state that they had received training pertaining to Asperger's syndrome. Then a teacher, Mrs. Lori Lee, when it was her turn to share her information, added, "I have no training with students like Jacob. I also have no experience working with students like Jacob. What I do have is a mother's heart for all my students. I will gladly get the training I need and love Jacob the whole way through this journey."

As the meeting progressed, our advocate asked what testing and services Jacob had received and was receiving. He rattled off each test that was required of children on the autism spectrum as well as the services that should be offered. We were surprised to learn that some of the required testing was never given or was overdue (the tests must be performed on a regular basis). Jacob also had not received some of the services required by law. The advocate's persistence in questioning, his knowledge of the laws and the rights of the student, and his endless quest for answers caused much tension in the meeting.

One by one, the advocate went through every single item on his list, addressing the school officials who could provide the answers. We heard a lot of apologies. *I'm not sure* and *I'll have to check into that* were offered up more than once. The process was so involved that we had to dismiss and meet again for a second and then a third time.

It was very expensive—extremely expensive—but it was all worth the money and the time because Jacob was tested, retested, and offered services that he desperately needed.

Before Jacob's annual ARD meeting the next year, the school asked if our advocate would be attending again. If so, the school said they would have their own advocate there too. Our advocate had put them through the wringer, and they had not enjoyed it. However, since we were satisfied with Jacob's progress at school, we felt like we did not need the advocate.

After resolving the indecent exposure incident, working through all the details of Jacob's ARD, and establishing the teamwork of using the tools Jacob was learning through behavior group, home, and school, Dariel and I finally believed everything was in place and that smooth sailing was ahead.

We were wrong.

More Challenges

During Jacob's second-grade year, his class went to the library as part of their regular rotation schedule. All of Jacob's teachers had been specifically taught that new situations were difficult for Jacob. His response to the rearranged lunchroom in first grade was a great example. The teachers were told that if you took Jacob and his class into any room outside their normal classroom, you could say to the students, "Go find a seat." But for Jacob, you would need to go to him and show him specifically where to sit. That simple action would alleviate his fear and anxiety.

Jacob's class entered the library and sat as they awaited instructions. The librarian told them to find a book they'd like to read. Everyone dispersed across the library to begin the hunt for a new book—everyone except Jacob. He had a meltdown because he was confused and didn't know what type of book to get. An entire school library full of possibilities was too overwhelming.

I wasn't aware this had happened until Jacob came home from school. As was my daily routine, I was going through his Behavior Notebook looking for check marks and reading through his homework list. An envelope with my name on it caught my attention. I opened it and began to read.

The librarian had written, "Mrs. Berry, I want to make you aware of a situation that occurred with Jacob today at school. His class was in the library, and they were instructed to go find a book. He had one of his episodes but was able to tell Mrs. Taylor (the vice principal) later that it was because he was confused about what to do. I had a library full of students and didn't really have the time to deal with him. I wanted you to know."

She "didn't have time to deal with him"? If she had taken five seconds to simply say to him, "Jacob, let me show you where to look for a book" or "Jacob, can I help you find a book?" the meltdown could have been avoided. She had been trained but would not be bothered to do what was asked to help a second grader.

I immediately called our advocate and read to him the note the librarian had written. "Can you believe her?"

He told me to write an official letter to the principal with two demands. Number one: The librarian must receive additional training on how to deal with Asperger's syndrome students and that training must be completed in the next six weeks. Number two: The librarian would apologize to me. He also encouraged me to file a complaint with the Texas Education Agency, but I decided against that. As a former teacher, I thought that was too harsh an action to take at that time. If there was another incident, then I would file the report. I did, however, include in the letter to the principal that

I would be contacting TEA if these two demands were not met.

I went in to see the principal the following morning after Jacob had gone to his classroom, handed her the letter, and told her I expected a response within the next forty-eight hours. I was contacted by the principal two days later; she told me the librarian was scheduled to receive the training I had asked for within the required time period and that I would be receiving a letter of apology from her. I received that letter the following day.

As pleased as I was that the situation had been resolved to my satisfaction, I was deeply discouraged that this incident had occurred after all the struggles and hard work we had put in. Dariel and I made it known that we were available anytime and would cooperate fully with the teachers and staff at the school. Our greatest desire was to see Jacob progress and improve with his social interactions. It was the first of many times that I felt we had taken three steps forward only to take one step back.

Unfortunately, the school was not the only place where we encountered problems.

Our church offered a program called AWANA where students in various age brackets memorized scripture. Jacob was in the SPARKS group when he was in second grade. One night during AWANA, all the students gathered in the church gym for a group activity. While I was standing in line with Jacob, an adult leader in Jacob's group approached me. I had never met her, but I could tell from the moment she started speaking that she was angry. I braced myself as she launched into a diatribe about Jacob's behavior. With all the disdain she could muster, she scolded me for allowing Jacob to behave badly in group. But what really agitated her was that the leaders never disciplined him or scolded him. She basically accused me of raising a horrible child and that I was a horrible parent because I never did anything about it.

I took a deep breath and bit my tongue to keep from going off on her. The tears that welled up from anger and frustration pooled in my eyes.

With a deep breath, I asked her, "Do you know what Asperger's syndrome is?"

"No, what is that?" She punctuated each word.

I informed her that it was a disorder on the autism spectrum that made social interaction difficult. As I was explaining the ways she could help Jacob, she interrupted me and said, "Well, it just sounds like a major excuse to me. All I know is something needs to be done about Jacob." She turned and stormed off.

I stood there, I'm not sure how long, totally stunned. There were adults and children all around me talking, laughing, and enjoying the group activities, but I stayed rooted in that one spot trying to absorb what had just transpired. Eventually, I pulled myself together and made a beeline for the children's pastor.

"Travis, do you know who that woman is?" I pointed to the lady who had just berated me and demeaned my son.

"Sure," he replied. "She's one of our group leaders."

I came closer to him, leaned in, and said, "I don't want her anywhere near Jacob, *ever*."

"Why?" Travis had grown very close to Jacob and knew about Asperger's syndrome and Jacob's struggles.

He was one of Jacob's biggest cheerleaders and encouragers. He was shocked when I told him what had happened and assured me that he would not allow her to be around Jacob and that he would talk to her.

Never before or after have I encountered such a vitriolic attitude toward my son.

How do nonbelievers make it through times like this without God? If he wasn't there and always available for me to vent my frustration to, express my fear and anger to, and ask forgiveness from when I think horrible thoughts about people who hurt the ones I love, I'd be a major mess.

Despite these painful incidents, Jacob was improving and had many more successes as he continued through elementary school. We were not done by any means, and we sure weren't going to give up.

6
GETTING SOMEWHERE

Commit to the Lord whatever you do, and he will establish your plans.

—Proverbs 16:3 (NIV)

Second Grade

The first day of second grade arrived, and we were ready. Prior to that first day, I had taken Jacob to Whispering Pines Elementary School to meet his teacher. She spent a few minutes getting to know him and showed him the ins and outs of her classroom. Knowing where the room was and what a typical day would look like plus the added bonus of meeting his new teacher all seemed to minimize Jacob's fear and anxiety.

Parents are allowed to walk their children into the classroom the first day, so Jacob and I arrived early that Monday morning. We were greeted by the principal, teachers who knew him from first grade, and some other students. There were familiar smiling faces everywhere as all the kids walked through the front door to begin a new year.

I was babbling words of encouragement as we made our way to his classroom, inwardly praying he'd be okay and not have any meltdowns.

We turned the corner and stood at the doorway of his classroom. He spotted his teacher across the room, and she gave him a big smile. But he turned back around for one last glimpse of Mom.

There it was. A jolting, devastating punch to the gut. Mrs. Kling had cautioned there would be moments like this, but I still wasn't prepared. The fear in his eyes was palpable, and I wanted to save him. I couldn't leave him there like that. But feet moving and heart breaking, I gave him one last hug and turned away. I had to. I had to let him go.

I walked slowly down the hall, fighting every maternal instinct within me. I somehow made it to the van. "God," I cried, "please, please be with Jacob. Be his peace, take away his fear. Be his strength."

We made it through the day with zero phone calls from the school. When Jacob climbed into the van after school, I said, "How did it go?"

"Good." And that was it. But, hey, I'll take a one-word response instead of a meltdown story any day of the week.

When I was driving Jacob to school one morning, our van's gas tank was almost on empty. Jacob noticed it from his seat and asked me before I dropped him off if I would be getting gas sometime that day. I assured him I would do just that. I drove up in front of Whispering Pines Elementary and watched him get out and walk in to start his day. That afternoon, I was waiting in the car line to pick him up when Mrs. Eastman approached my car and asked me to roll down my window.

She peered in at me and asked, "Mrs. Berry, did you need gas this morning?"

"Yes, I did. How did you know?"

"Mrs. Berry, let me just tell you right now that *anytime* you need to get gas, please do. I will never count Jacob tardy if you need to stop on the way to school and fill up."

I started to laugh. "Oh no! What happened?"

Mrs. Eastman informed me that Jacob had been distracted all morning. His teacher didn't understand why he was acting so strangely until he told her that he was worried about me because our car was almost out of gas. Even after the teacher reassured him, Jacob continued to worry throughout the day.

I promised the principal that I would never again bring Jacob to school without having plenty of fuel in my gas tank.

Jacob's second-grade year went smoothly, the only hiccup being the incident with the librarian. He faithfully attended the weekly behavior group and once again carried the Behavior Notebook with him throughout the day, seeking those wonderful check marks from every teacher. I'm happy to report that he received many more in the second grade than in the first grade.

One night at Behavior Plus, after the parental observation time, the group dismissed, and Mrs. Kling waved me over to where she was sitting.

"I can tell you and Dariel have really been working with Jacob," she said.

I was excited to hear that, but I asked, "Why?"

She replied, "Tonight was a rough one for Jacob. He didn't receive as many tickets as he wanted." (The students received tickets as a reward throughout the session and were able to exchange them for prizes at the end of the group meeting.) "He didn't get to go first to select a prize, and the prize he wanted was taken by someone else. I was worried that he might have a meltdown, but at the end of our session, Jacob threw his hand up in the air and pronounced proudly, 'I am handling my disappointment!'"

I smiled a *really* big smile.

Mrs. Kling continued. "Julie, that wouldn't have happened a few weeks ago. Jacob would have gone into a full-blown meltdown when everything went so wrong. But he was right. He handled it, and I know that's because of the work you and Dariel are doing with him at home."

Mrs. Kling was absolutely correct. It was hard work, but Dariel and I constantly applied what Jacob was learning at Behavior Plus to his actions at school, at home, and at church. This consistency produced the overwhelming improvement.

Also in second grade, Jacob began weekly sessions with a special education teacher who had a huge impact on his growth. It was Mrs. Lori Lee, the same teacher who had impressed us with her openness and honesty in the first ARD meeting with our advocate. One day when Jacob's group was walking in the hall, Mrs. Lee fussed at one of the students who was not staying in line. As soon as she finished rebuking the child, Jacob stopped in his tracks and wouldn't budge. No matter how much Mrs. Lee cajoled and pleaded with him, he would not say a word or move a muscle. Jacob was in full shutdown. Eventually, Jacob rejoined the class, and Mrs. Lee asked him what had caused the shutdown. He was able to articulate to her that she scared him because of the tone of voice she used with the boy who had gotten out of line.

Although Jacob experienced another shutdown, his recovery was much quicker than it had been in the past, and he was able to clearly express to Mrs. Lee what had caused his reaction.

Progress! And that word pretty much sums up second grade. Life wasn't perfect, but Jacob was coping better with change and fear. Superflex was in attack mode fighting off Rock Brain and Glass Man. Victories weren't 100 percent, but they were occurring at a much steadier pace.

Third Grade

Transitioning to third grade was even smoother. Jacob met with his teacher, Mrs. Vincent, before school, and their initial time together was amazing. After she showed Jacob around her classroom and pointed out Jacob's desk, they sat down and had a conversation. My son, who so often feared new circumstances and interactions, talked about his summer, visiting with his grandparents, swimming, going on vacation, and on and on. He then shared some of the techniques he had learned at Behavior Plus and the ones he thought were most helpful. He told her about expected and unexpected behavior, the full or empty cup, and Superflex. It was a great first step, and I was extremely proud.

Jacob still had to keep his Behavior Notebook, and he continued practicing the strategies he learned at weekly behavior group. Parents were no longer required to observe the last part of his group sessions at Behavior Plus. It was now Jacob's responsibility to let his dad and me know what activities he had participated in and what he had learned. The meltdowns and shutdowns were steadily decreasing, but he still struggled with participating in new activities and games in physical education class, although the coaches were great at coming up with ways to help him overcome his fears. That often involved letting Dariel and me know about the new activity ahead of time so we could practice with him and prepare him. Other times, the teacher found an alternative activity that Jacob could easily master.

One of the primary strategies implemented by Mrs. Vincent in the classroom was to remove the element of surprise as much as possible from Jacob's day. For example, if Mrs. Vincent knew she was going to miss a day of school, she took time to let Jacob know she would be gone and who the substitute would be. If the school followed a different schedule for the day or altered the normal routine in any way, she would inform Jacob beforehand.

One of our favorite things that Mrs. Vincent implemented for Jacob was the use of social stories. Social stories are short, sometimes illustrated descriptions of a particular event or activity that includes specific information about what to expect in a situation.

Here are some examples of the stories Mrs. Vincent used with Jacob.

EXAMPLE #1:

Field Day Social Story for Friday, May 23, 2008

This Friday, all third graders get to participate in the field day.

In the morning, we are going to walk into the cafeteria with our flags for the opening ceremony.

Then we will come back to class.

We will all get to go outside and do the tug-of-war and water balloon toss.

After that, we will get a cool treat and eat snow cones.

Our sack lunches will be eaten in the classroom.

After lunch, we will start the events for the field day outside.

We will travel to all the different stations and complete all the events.

If our class does not win an event, it is okay as long as we try our best and work as a team.

Once we are finished with all the events, we will go inside the cafeteria and have the closing ceremony with the awards.

We will not be switching classes today, and you will be with Mrs. Vincent all day.
We will not go to recess or specials today.

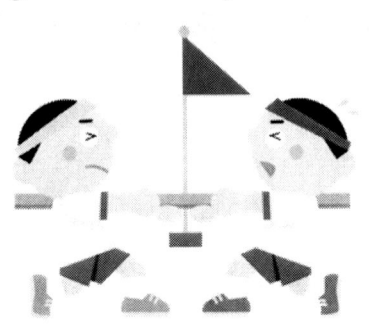

EXAMPLE #2:

Field Trip Social Story for Friday, May 9, 2008

This Friday, all third graders get to go on a field trip.
First, we are going to get ready and put our lunches in a cooler.
When the buses arrive, we are going to line up to get on the bus.
We will ride the bus to the Houston Museum of Natural Science.
Once we arrive, we will line up to enter the IMAX theater.
It will be a very large auditorium with students from other schools.
When the movie gets ready to start, the room will get dark, and we will have to be quiet.
A person will speak on the loud speaker to review the rules that we must follow.

GETTING SOMEWHERE

After the IMAX show, we will take a short bathroom break.
Then we will enter the planetarium to see *Starry Night*.
The planetarium will also become dark, and we will follow the same rules that we did in the IMAX theater.
After the show, we will leave the museum and get back on the bus.
We will ride the bus to Independence Park in Pearland for lunch.
At the park, we will eat our sack lunches and then play.
Then we will ride the bus back to school.

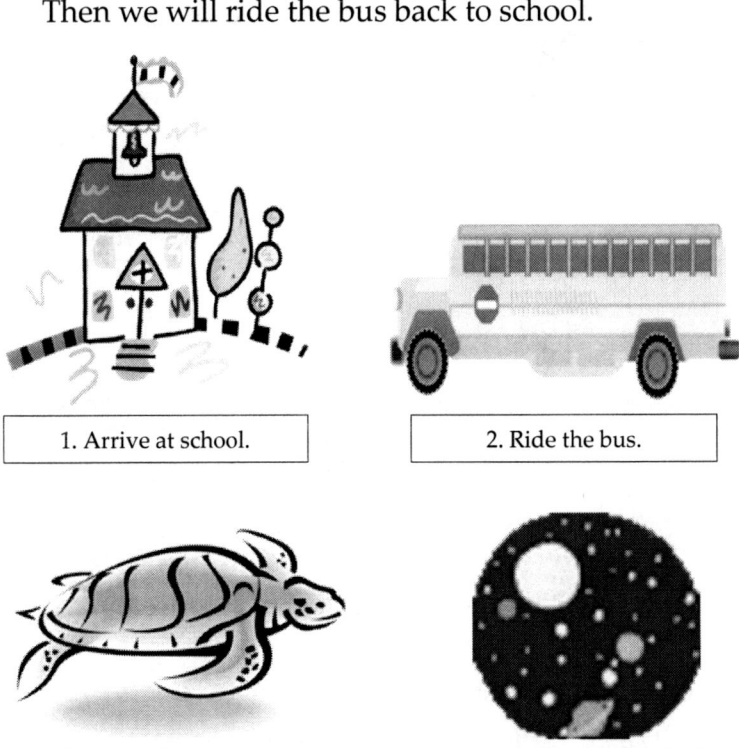

1. Arrive at school.

2. Ride the bus.

3. Watch the IMAX.

4. Watch the planetarium.

WHY DO I HAVE ASPERGER'S?

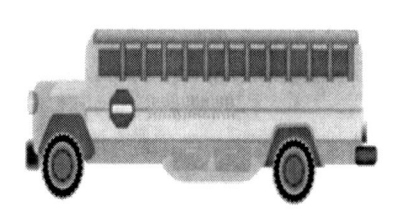

| 5. Ride the bus to the park. | 6. Eat lunch. |

| 7. Ride the bus back to school. | 8. Arrive back at Whispering Pines. |

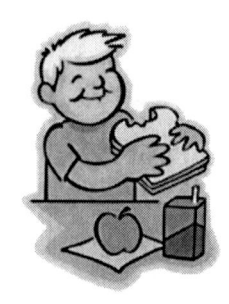

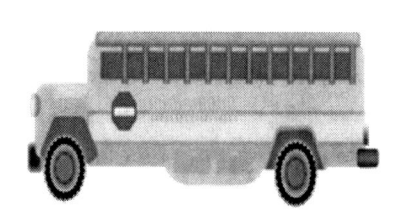

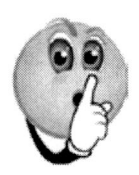

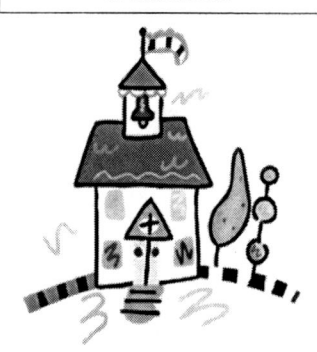

EXAMPLE #3:

TAKS Social Story for Wednesday, March 5, 2008

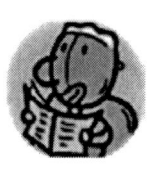

I am a third grader.
Third graders have to take the reading TAKS test.
Wednesday, I will take the TAKS test for reading.
When I get to school, I will come to Mrs. Vincent's classroom to get my things ready for the day.
I will need pencils and books to read.
Mrs. Vincent will give me an index card to use if I want to.

I cannot write anything on my index card.

I can eat my snack and drink water anytime during the test as long as I scoot my chair away from my desk so I won't spill anything on my test booklet.

I will be with Ms. Cole today to take the test.

I will not go to Ms. Pearson's class today.

I will still have lunch with my class.

I have to be very quiet during and after taking the test.

If I have a question or need help, I can raise my hand.

If I need to go to the bathroom or get up, I must raise my hand and get permission.

When I am finished with the test, I need to raise my hand to turn it in after I have done my two-finger check.

After I turn in my test, I can only read a book or put my head on my desk.

I will not have specials or recess today.

Mrs. Vincent sent these social stories home with Jacob prior to the event so we could reinforce what she was doing. They were such great tools in alleviating Jacob's anxiety.

Jacob and the Bee

Jacob has always been a great speller. I asked him once what his secret was, and he told me that once he sees a word, he can memorize how to spell it.

When Riley was in third grade, he used to sit at the kitchen table after supper so Dariel or I could call out his spelling words for him to spell back to us. Jacob usually sat at the kitchen table too, working on his homework. On occasion, Riley misspelled a word, and before Dariel and I could correct him, Jacob did the job for us. Jacob never spelled a word incorrectly. Riley wasn't too happy about it, but Jacob thought it was great.

In third grade, Mrs. Vincent selected Jacob to be one of only two students to represent the third grade in the school spelling bee. Although my husband and I were thrilled that Jacob had received this honor, we also privately experienced mild hysteria.

I shared my concerns with Dariel. "A spelling bee? In front of the whole school? Oh my!"

"I know," he said. "What do we do? Do we let him get up there?"

We both experienced flashbacks to the now less frequent but ever so disturbing crying fits, the screaming, the flinging himself on the floor. Even the slightest possibility of that happening on a stage in front of the whole school was cause for panic.

Jacob had his weekly behavior group meeting the day after we were informed of the upcoming spelling bee. When group concluded and the children exited the room, my husband and I asked Jacob to wait in the lobby so we could speak with Mrs. Kling.

Jacob had told her about the spelling bee, and she was beaming with pride on his behalf.

Dariel and I looked at each other, and I asked, somewhat incredulously, "You think we should allow him to do it?"

"Absolutely!" she replied without any hesitation.

"But what if, what if—"

"Julie, you *have* to let Jacob do this. He's ready, and you can't put him in a protective bubble all his life. You've got to let him get up on that stage, and if he falls, he just falls. This is part of his growth."

I looked at my husband. We both knew she was exactly right. We both knew we needed to let Jacob go out on his own.

"Okay, we'll do it."

Parenting isn't for cowards.

Dariel and I practiced with Jacob daily, encouraging him and doing our best to prepare him in every way.

When the big day arrived, Dariel, Riley, and I sat on the front row, ready to cheer Jacob on. I could see him on the stage. His body language was screaming, "I'm scared!" We collectively held our breaths as Jacob stood up to spell his first word.

Yes! He spelled his first word correctly and returned to his seat. This continued a few more rounds until Jacob came forward again and was asked to spell *knapsack*. When the letter *n* was the first letter to come out of his mouth, I knew he would be disqualified. When he completed misspelling the word, my husband and I tensed as we awaited his reaction.

Nothing. Jacob calmly took his seat and waited until the bee was completed.

Has any other parent ever been so proud when their child did *not* win the spelling bee? To this day, I find it difficult to retell this amazing day in Jacob's life without shedding a few tears. What a monumental achievement this was in his young life and his journey through Asperger's syndrome!

That scared little boy who once walked into a cafeteria and ran out in tears because the tables were rearranged got up on that stage, faced down his fears, and sat down with dignity when he was eliminated. In the grand scheme of the Berry family, that was more of a victory than any trophy Jacob could have ever won.

More from Behavior Plus

Jacob continued to learn many things at Behavior Plus, such as idioms. An idiom is defined as "a group of words established by usage as having a meaning not deductible from those of the individual words." Here are two examples of idioms: "It's raining cats and dogs" and "She got up on the wrong side of the bed." Since people with Asperger's syndrome are very literal, the coaches at Behavior Plus spent several group sessions discussing different idioms and helping the students understand their meanings.

One of my favorite behaviors Jacob learned while attending Behavior Plus was this: "Don't yuck someone else's yum." In other words, when offered food, even new food, in a social setting, you need to try at least one bite.

This was another one: "Just because you think it, doesn't mean you have to say it." That's like the time Jacob's pediatrician, who was advanced in age, walked into the exam room, and Jacob proclaimed, "You're old!"

He also learned this: "Was funny once." Jacob and those in his group had the habit of repeating a comment over and over when that comment had caused others to laugh. They repeated it, hoping to cause more laughter. We used "Was funny once" in our family many times — and not just for Jacob.

Behavior group also taught the students simple things like saying thank you when given a gift, and to blend in, meaning not to engage in behavior or actions that singled you out among your peers.

It was so impressive to see Jacob implement everything he was learning. He absorbed every bit of it and diligently put it into practice.

Fourth Grade

When fourth grade arrived, Jacob once again met his teacher and toured his classroom prior to the first day of school. He was still required to carry his Behavior Notebook to every class and receive check marks for expected behavior. On the second day of school, Jacob, on his own initiative, approached his teacher and asked to stop carrying the Behavior Notebook. He explained to her that he was learning at behavior group the need to blend in, and since no other student in fourth grade was required to carry a Behavior Notebook, he wasn't blending in. His teacher agreed, and the Behavior Notebook went away, never to be seen again.

When Jacob came home that day, he told me what had happened with the notebook and then simply walked away and up the stairs to the game room.

I was dumbstruck. *What just happened? He did what? On his own?*

In fourth grade, Jacob was allowed to take the state required standardized tests with his classmates. Every year before that, he had the test administered to him in a separate room because he tended to hum and sing to himself, which, of course, distracted others. Behavior Plus and blending in had taught him to keep that in check, so now he no longer needed those special accommodations.

One of those standardized tests was a writing test. A couple months after he had completed the test, Jacob's teacher was contacted by test officials. They were concerned that someone other than Jacob had written the essay on his test. He scored so high that the officials thought there might be something amiss. The school and teacher assured the test officials that everything had been done according to mandated guidelines and that Jacob was just that talented at writing.

This is the essay Jacob wrote for that test in fourth grade:

> "B-O-C-K! B-O-C-K!" I was acting like a big chicken. My family and I were waiting in line to ride the Loco Rio! It was as long as a country mile. You can't believe how surprising it was to get myself in such fun and chaos! Here's the whole story.
>
> "When are we going to get our turn?" I moaned. It felt like we've been waiting for hours to finally have our chance to get on the ride. After a very long time of waiting it was our turn. "Yes!" I hollered. All this time of waiting will finally pay off. I jumped into a giant inner-tube. I took the seat next to my mom. "Momma's boy," Riley sighed. I gazed back at him and rolled my eyes. The ride started. I was a little nervous. All of a sudden I started to shake. We were going down a conveyor belt into the water. P-L-O-P!

We were lazily floating along. The first thing I spotted was a bundle of water squirters! I tried my best to dodge them. I leaned back in my seat as far as I could. One shot hit my big brother Riley in the face. "Bullseye!" I bellowed. Then I started to crack up. One squirt nearly hit my little brother Keaton, but Riley blocked it off! "Thanks," declared Keaton. We got past the water squirters. "Phew!" I blurted, but little did I know the second obstacle was a humongous WATERFALL! "Aaah!" I screamed. B-O-C-K!

B-O-C-K! I felt like that chicken again. The waterfall was spewing out gallons of water. My eyes got as big as lemons. This really surprised me! The inner-tube's speed went up. Good bye life, I thought. The inner-tube made a curve, and I was directly under the fall. S-P-L-A-S-H! Brrr! The water was icy. I looked like a drowned rat. Oh, well, at least I don't have to take a shower tonight, I thought. We went up another conveyor belt, and the ride ended.

"Awesome!" I shouted. I wanted to ride the Loco Rio again, but I overheard my mom say no when Riley asked to. Bummer, I thought. Oh, well, at least I can come next year. The surprising thrill of the ride woke me up. I will always enjoy the Loco Rio.

Then came the traditional all-night fourth-grade slumber party. Dariel and I were concerned. Jacob had a sleepover in first grade, but he came home during the night after having a tantrum because he couldn't figure out how to unzip his sleeping bag. There had never been another sleepover except with family members. But as we learned in the spelling bee, we knew we had to allow him to go. He made it through the entire night without incident and had a great time.

One of my favorite memories from Jacob's fourth-grade year was a homework assignment using the dictionary. I was upstairs putting away laundry, and Jacob was downstairs at the kitchen table having very little success at completing the assignment. The teacher had instructed the students to look up words in the dictionary from a list she had provided and write the definition beside the word. Jacob didn't understand how to look words up and had gone into a total shutdown.

I could hear my husband encouraging him. "Come on, Jacob. Don't let Rock Brain win. Be Superflex and stop this shutdown." This went for several minutes as Dariel tried desperately to get through to Jacob.

Suddenly I had an idea. I marched down the stairs, sat down beside Jacob, and got him to look at me.

"Jacob, you know you have Asperger's syndrome, right?"

"Yeah."

"So, do you know that people with Asperger's syndrome have a lot of fear when trying something new? Your dad and I could get this same assignment and be a little nervous because we weren't exactly sure what to do, but we would go ahead and try. But Asperger's syndrome is causing you to be so afraid that you'll be wrong that you're scared to even attempt it. You've come a long way and learned so much. Don't let this beat you. You're smart, and you can do it."

He looked at me and opened the dictionary. We showed him how to do the first word, and he was off to the races. A few minutes later, my husband and I sat down to watch something on TV in the living room, which was adjacent to the kitchen. Every few minutes Jacob said, "Hey, listen to this word," and he read a word and the definition. Dariel and I looked at each other after several minutes of this and said, "Is this the same kid who was in full shutdown a few minutes ago?" The change was remarkable.

I believe that God gave me the words to speak to Jacob, because on my own, I had no idea my approach would be successful. But Jacob was older, and some of the young, child-centered strategies weren't working. He'd grown old enough to know about Asperger's syndrome and its characteristics, and being reminded of that helped him overcome.

Gone but Never Forgotten

As Jacob's fourth-grade year came to a close, his time at Whispering Pines Elementary School ended. Middle school was next. I couldn't help but marvel at what had taken place the last four years. The progress from those excruciating first few months to where we were now seemed unthinkable.

One day during the final week of school, I sat in the car line waiting to pick up Jacob. As I moved my van forward in the line, the principal approached and motioned for me to roll down my window.

"I want you to know something," she said. "Since Jacob's enrollment here in first grade, the training our staff has received and our success with him and students like him have given us quite the reputation in the community. Just today, I met with two separate families that are going to sell their current homes so they can purchase a new home that is zoned to Whispering Pines. They want their children to attend here so we can provide them with the help they need."

Tears filled my eyes.

A few years after Jacob left Whispering Pines Elementary, as I was beginning to write this book, I interviewed the principal and some of Jacob's former teachers. Every one of them, without exception, told me that working with Jacob changed his or her life for the better.

One teacher wrote, "The experiences I've had with Jacob have made me a better Christian, mother, advocate, teacher, and friend." Another stated, "I think that not only did Jacob grow and improve, but he helped me grow and improve as a teacher. He opened my eyes to teaching in different ways. He taught me patience and how to approach a student with Asperger's. He was my first student officially diagnosed with Asperger's, and my experiences with him have taught me more than I could have ever expected. When he walked through my classroom on the first day of school, he not only opened my eyes to how to work effectively with him, but also how to work effectively with all the future students that I would have."

This young, frightened little boy who'd entered Whispering Pines Elementary at the age of six and struggled so much was an inspiration to all by showing those around him that anything is possible and that not all children are the same.

I think that makes me the most thankful to God. What some would see as a burden or hindrance is instead a special child who touched the hearts of numerous people and impacted their lives for the better.

The elementary years had seen amazing progress, but we weren't finished yet.

7
LEAPS AND BOUNDS

The steadfast love of the LORD never ceases; his mercies never come to an end; they are new every morning; great is your faithfulness.

—Lamentations 3:22–23

Middle School

I'm embarrassed to admit that I was *that* parent. The first day of middle school arrived, and I went in with Jacob through the front doors. Very quickly I was approached by a friendly staff member who kindly informed me that parents did not walk their students into middle school.

Sheepishly, I gave Jacob a final word of encouragement and made my way out to the van.

As we entered the middle school years, the meltdowns were subsiding and occurred very rarely. The shutdowns, however, still reared their ugly heads. Whenever Jacob received an assignment he didn't understand, he sat at his desk, making no attempt to do the work. Fortunately, since the teachers all had access to Jacob's IEP, they were aware that his actions were not a disobedience issue.

With every shutdown, Dariel and I talked with him, reminding him that he knew how to ask for help. There were days when he was able to do that, but there were still times when he succumbed to the shutdown.

In addition to emphasizing the tools he'd learned in behavior group, Dariel and I also took away privileges such as his Nintendo DS as a motivation to stop the shutdowns. Since he was older, this technique was very effective.

On occasion throughout Jacob's middle school years, I received an email or note from one of his teachers. They detailed a particular assignment that Jacob didn't complete. Initially, I asked Jacob to see what the issue was. Although I had expectations that something outside the norm had occurred, without fail, it was always because he didn't understand the assignment.

One afternoon, I went into the office at the middle school to pick up Jacob a few minutes early. As I waited for him to arrive, the assistant principal, Mrs. Finch, approached me.

"Oh, Mrs. Berry. I'm glad I saw you," she said. "I need to talk to you. Jacob hasn't completed an assignment in math, and his teacher wanted me to check with you and ask what you thought the problem might—"

She was interrupted as Jacob walked into the office.

Without allowing her to complete her sentence, I said, "Jacob, Mrs. Finch says you haven't turned in your math assignment. It's because you don't understand what to do, correct?"

Jacob nodded.

"Jacob, if you don't complete that assignment by tonight, you cannot have your DS until the weekend. Do you understand? You know your father and I expect you to ask for help when you are confused about work the teacher requires, don't you?"

"Yes, ma'am. I'll get it done."

With that taken care of, I turned my attention back to the assistant principal. She stood there, mouth open, gaping at us.

I thanked her for letting me know about Jacob, and we walked out of the office as she continued to stand rooted in the same spot.

Recounting the story to my husband later, I could only assume that Mrs. Finch had a totally different expectation of what would take place, having been conditioned to hear parents make excuses for their children or children denying the accusation, blaming the teacher or generally having a bad attitude. My blunt, to-the-point conversation with Jacob about what we expected, his willing attitude, and compliance dumbfounded her. I will never forget the look on her face.

Except for that interesting exchange, the two years Jacob spent in middle school as he completed fifth and sixth grade were pretty routine. To this day, if I happen to be at that middle school working with the band students or teaching a private lesson, teachers and staff who knew Jacob stop and ask me how he's doing. His life continued to impact those around him.

Life outside of School

School wasn't the only place we saw great progress with Jacob. Remembering that any new situation caused Jacob to panic, Dariel and I were thrilled to see him asking questions and being proactive when entering new situations.

One Sunday while Jacob was in fifth grade, our church had a guest group come in to lead everything from the worship service to caring for babies in the nursery to the children's ministry. The special day had been advertised for several weeks prior, so Jacob was aware that there would be something new and different.

On Saturday night, Jacob came to me and said, "Mom, what exactly is going to be happening tomorrow at church?"

"I'm not sure," I replied. "I've never attended any event with this group, so I really have no idea."

He just stood there. Then it dawned on me. He was asking about the children's service because he knew this new group would be in charge of the children's area where he would be in attendance.

"Oh, you're asking about what they'll be doing with the kids, right?"

"Yes, I just want to know what will be going on."

"I understand. You know what? We'll just ask them. How does that sound?"

He voiced his approval and walked out of the room.

I did the happy dance. Jacob didn't want to be afraid. He was planning and preparing for change.

The next morning, Jacob and I walked into the large room at church where the guest leaders were setting up the children's area and welcoming the kids who had already arrived. I spotted someone who looked like she was in charge, grabbed Jacob's hand, and approached her.

"Hi. This is Jacob. He's my son, and he has Asperger's syndrome. It would be really helpful if you could explain to him exactly what's going to happen in here today."

"Of course!" she replied and offered up a big smile. She focused her attention on Jacob and gave him a minute-by-minute schedule of the morning's program. When she finished, I looked at Jacob and said, "Does that help? Are you good to go?"

He smiled and said yes. After watching him take a seat beside his brother Keaton, I headed into the sanctuary, pleased as I could be about what I had just witnessed. We were definitely getting somewhere.

The summer after sixth grade, we experienced another huge life event. Over the years, our family has seen many movies together. My husband, Riley, Keaton, and I have similar tastes when it comes to movies. We love action and sci-fi with lots of loud music and dazzling special effects. Jacob? Not so much. He's more of a *Diary of a Wimpy Kid* or *Despicable Me* kind of guy.

When he was too young to stay home by himself, he begrudgingly came along and sat through many a movie he couldn't have cared less about. But he was now twelve years old, and when I asked him about going to see our most recent movie selection, he said, "I don't want to go.

I'll stay home by myself." He had witnessed Riley stay at home alone before and figured he was now old enough to do the same.

Gulp! *Don't react,* I told myself. "Okay," I said. "Are you sure?"

Not missing a beat, he looked up from his Nintendo DS and said, "Yeah."

"Dariel!" I yelled as soon as I left Jacob's room.

"Yes?" he answered from downstairs.

"Come up to our bedroom, please."

He marched up the stairs and entered the bedroom. I closed the door.

"Jacob doesn't want to go to the movie," I said as Dariel sat down on the bed to put on his shoes. "He's . . . uh . . . well, he's going to stay home alone."

He stopped tying his shoe lace and looked up. "No."

"Why not?" I knew exactly why not.

"He cannot stay home alone."

"I know, I know. It's Jacob," I said. "But he's the same age Riley was when we left him alone for the first time. We've told him he can do anything. So, do we really believe that or has that just been lip service?"

"You're right," he replied. "It's just hard."

Yes, it was.

We called Jacob into the room and carefully rehearsed what to do in case of an emergency, how to work the alarm, and how long we'd be gone, all the while trying to sound normal.

I texted him several times during the movie, and there were no issues. We returned home a couple of hours later to find him right where we left him. To Jacob, it was no big deal. To Mom and Dad, it was huge. Another milestone successfully completed.

Another example of progress in middle school came with Jacob's stuffed animals. Jacob loves stuffed animals. He had gathered quite a collection over the years—lots of bears, a frog, a leopard, a tiger, a shark, a caterpillar, a raccoon, a turtle, an eagle, a rabbit, puppies, and many other variations of the animal kingdom with a few Pokémons thrown in. He had a name for each one and could tell you when he received it.

The animals—all of them—took up residence in Jacob's bed. We occasionally discussed perhaps releasing some of them into the wild, but I never pushed the issue.

The summer after sixth grade, when Jacob was twelve, I walked up the stairs one afternoon to start a load of laundry. Jacob stepped out of his bedroom and said, "Mom, I moved my animals."

I put down the laundry basket and walked over to look at his bed. Sure enough, there they all were in a neatly arranged pile on the floor at the foot of Jacob's bed. (His one holdout was a bear his grandparents had given him when he was about six months old. His name was Banana Bear, and he still sleeps with Jacob to this day.)

I was stunned. I had often imagined Jacob explaining to his fiancée that she would be sharing their marital bed with him and thirty of his closest friends.

A menagerie of companions who had been with Jacob through bad dreams, sick days, thunderstorms, late night bedtime stories, and family prayer times now lay on his floor in all their glorious, stuffed, colorful splendor. Without an ultimatum from his parents, without tears or a meltdown, with no prompting whatsoever, my son with Asperger's syndrome had made a huge decision by himself that forever changed his way of life as he had always known it.

That morning, Jacob had woken up snuggling with all his childhood friends. That night, he would go to bed with only one. Jacob was definitely maturing and continuing to progress.

Break a Leg

Jacob's seventh-grade year was off to a great start. He and I went to the junior high two days before school started and met with his counselor. She answered several questions and, using Jacob's schedule, walked us through the school so he could locate each of his classrooms. Once we were done, Jacob took the schedule and walked the route by himself, finding each of his rooms without difficulty.

As in middle school, meltdowns were a thing of the past, but we continued to deal with the occasional shutdown as Jacob faced class assignments he didn't understand. Then our neatly packaged little world was broken—literally.

Just forty-eight hours after Jacob officially became a teenager, on a rainy Saturday in February, our family experienced a day never to be forgotten.

Jacob and Riley attended a weekend church camp. They left on Friday to spend two nights with other youth at a retreat about 40 minutes away.

We received the call on Saturday afternoon.

All the campers had gone on a treasure hunt out in the woods. While hunting, Jacob had slipped in the mud and fallen. He was complaining about his leg and refusing to get up because of the pain. We learned later that when Jacob slipped, his leg bent backward underneath him.

We were concerned, but in all transparency, Dariel and I just thought he was in the middle of a shutdown and were more annoyed than anything else. Dariel drove to the camp to check on him, and during that time, the church leaders managed to lift Jacob up onto a golf cart and drive him back to the main building.

Dariel arrived home with Jacob and helped him onto the nearest couch. We looked at his leg but didn't see any obvious trauma—no blood, no bones protruding from the skin. Remembering the whole leg pain incident back in kindergarten, which included two hospital visits and an ambulance ride, we were hesitant about how to proceed. And Jacob wasn't crying or complaining about any intense pain. He just said, "It hurts."

We called a friend of ours who is a registered nurse. She came right over, examined the leg, and told us to take him to the hospital immediately. With the whole family in tow, we ended up at a hospital in the medical center in Houston, Texas. The doctor informed us that the breaks (notice I said *breaks*—plural) were so severe that Jacob required surgery as soon as possible.

By the time Jacob was admitted, examined, X-rayed, and seen by the doctor, it was after midnight. Dariel stayed while I took Riley and Keaton home to get some sleep.

Before I left the emergency room, I told Jacob I'd be back later. He was casually lying on a gurney out in the hall playing on his Nintendo DS and being his humorous self with anyone who walked by. He wasn't crying or screaming or displaying any signs of distress despite the fact that his tibia and fibula were broken.

Leaving Riley in charge, I rose early and headed back to the hospital the next morning. I sent Dariel home to shower and rest. Jacob had been taken into surgery. A couple of hours later, the nurse escorted me to the recovery room where Jacob lay, groggy and still holding onto Banana Bear, with a huge green cast covering his right leg.

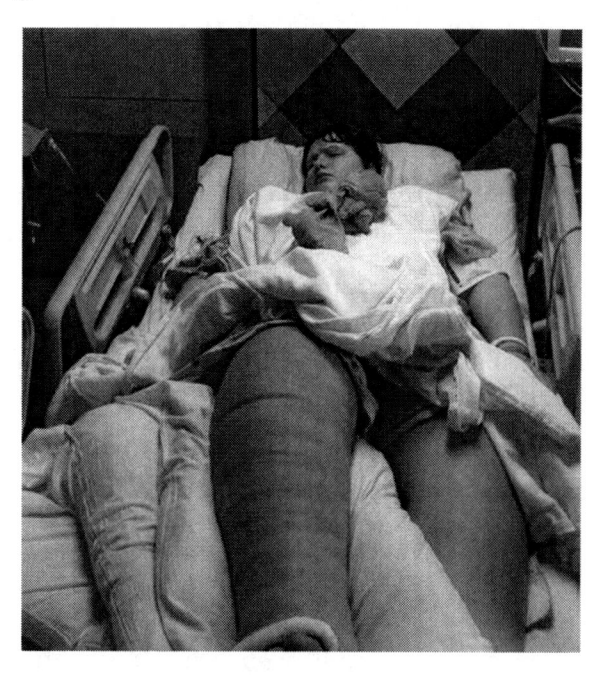

After two days in the hospital, Jacob returned home and took up residence in our downstairs recliner. The living room was his home for the next few months. Fortunately, we had a downstairs half bath that we equipped with side rails and a raised toilet seat. We also had to purchase a walker and a cane and rent a wheelchair. My living room looked like a hospital room had thrown up in it.

That large green cast was so heavy that it took two people to lift it so Jacob could go to the bathroom. A few days after the surgery, he was still in extreme pain, especially in his right ankle. We were counting down until the next time he saw the pediatric orthopedic surgeon, Dr. Monroe.

Ten days after Jacob's surgery, an X-ray at his checkup showed that the bones in his leg were moving and that his pain was caused by the ankle bone attempting to shift to one side. The surgeon informed us that he needed another surgery.

Jacob and I arrived at the hospital at 5:30 a.m. the next morning. After checking in, we waited patiently for someone to wheel him into surgery. Jacob's youth pastor called and prayed with him over the phone. Then a nurse appeared and spoke briefly to Jacob before wheeling him back to be prepped for surgery.

Dariel and I had taught Jacob as he grew older that he needed to communicate with any doctor or medical professional before having a procedure. Because so much anxiety for people with Asperger's syndrome is wrapped in the unknown, we trained him to tell others that he had Asperger's syndrome and would appreciate being informed of what was going to happen because he doesn't like surprises. He had already done this at appointments with the dental hygienist and his general practitioner.

I was so proud as I observed his interaction with the hospital staff while they prepared him for surgery. He asked numerous questions, and, being Jacob, he threw in some jokes and funny comments along the way.

As they came to roll his gurney into surgery, I had a flashback to when Jacob was nine months old and a nurse came and took him from my arms to have tubes put in his ears. It was so very hard to let go of him then, and I didn't find it one bit easier now.

I knew it could be hours, but every time the door of the waiting area opened, I looked up expectantly, hoping to see Jacob's surgeon. Hours felt like days as I waited and prayed and waited and prayed.

Finally, Dr. Monroe appeared. "The surgery went great," he said. "There was more damage than I thought. We had to put a plate in one break and pins in the other. I believe the leg will begin to heal correctly now."

I could not believe the extent of hardware in Jacob's leg when we saw his X-rays.

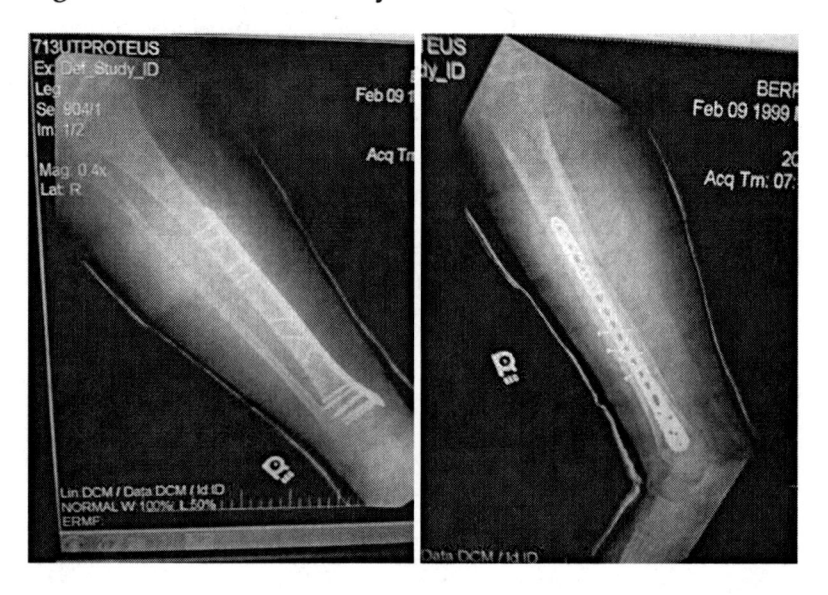

I thanked Dr. Monroe, received some post-op instructions, and finally joined Jacob in recovery. Once again, his treasured Banana Bear was close by.

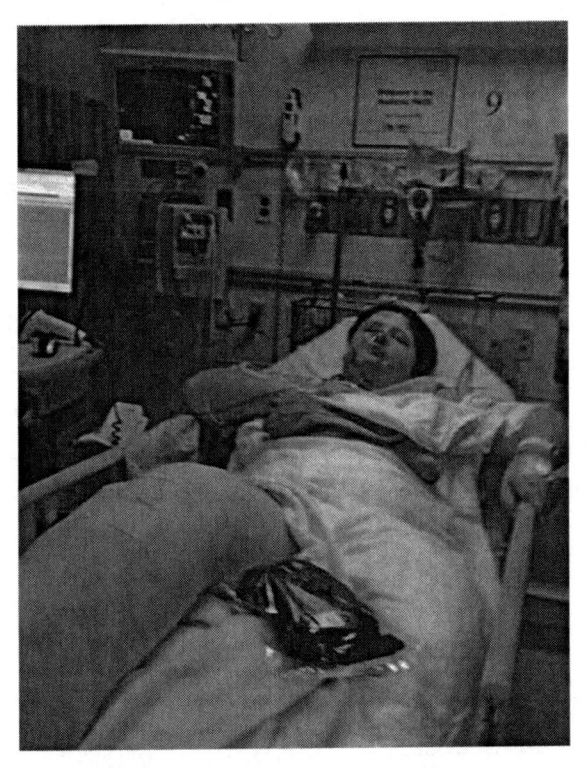

When Jacob began to wake up, he complained of intense pain. The nurses administered medication and moved him to a hospital room to begin another forty-eight-hour stay.

About two hours after the nurse settled him into his room, a physical therapist stopped by.

I thought he was just going to introduce himself, but I was wrong. Despite my hesitance and Jacob's outright insistence that he wasn't ready, the therapist made Jacob sit up in bed. With the use of a walker, he guided Jacob into the bathroom and then back to bed. Before the therapist even left the hospital room, Jacob was crying because of the profound pain.

I called the nurse who promised to come as soon as she could to administer additional pain medication. Although it seemed like an eternity, the nurse was true to her word, and within five minutes she was in the room pushing the meds through Jacob's IV.

By that point, however, Jacob was inconsolable. I held him as he sobbed. His cries were like that of a wounded animal. I prayed for him and whispered words of comfort in his ear. It seemed like forever, but mercifully, the pain medication kicked in, and he was able to get some rest.

As soon as my husband arrived, I was out the door and heading for the nurse's station. I demanded to know the name of the physical therapist and told the head nurse what had happened. She listened to my concerns, agreed with me, and we never saw that physical therapist again during Jacob's time in the hospital.

The whole incident was so traumatic for Jacob that when the new physical therapist came to work with him the next day, Jacob initially refused to cooperate. But Dariel talked him through it, and once Jacob was up and moving, he was actually excited.

Looking back, it is amazing to realize that the physical therapist incident was the only time during this whole incident that Jacob crumbled. He'd fractured his leg severely in two places out in the woods. He was loaded into a golf cart and then transported home. He went to an emergency room where he was placed on a gurney for hours awaiting surgery. He had the first surgery, came home, took up residence in a recliner, and had to have assistance to even move. Now, he'd endured a second surgery where pins and a plate where placed in his leg. Even though he had wrestled with fear, frustration, and impatience, he met every obstacle head-on with lots of humor mixed in, exhibiting a strength I never knew was possible from the same child who spent the first part of his life having horrendous meltdowns.

Jacob returned home and settled in his recliner. He was placed in the homebound program at school because of the extent of his injury and because the doctor had put him on blood thinners, which restricted his activities (blood clots were a possibility).

An ARD was required to officially begin the homebound period. I arrived at the ARD meeting, expecting compassion and understanding for Jacob's condition. Unfortunately, money seemed to be the priority rather than the welfare of the child.

The woman leading the ARD session interrogated me. "There's no way Jacob can come to school?" she asked.

"Well, sure if you want to hire someone to push him around in a wheelchair."

She considered the option. "That might be possible."

"Well, then you're going to have to hire a nurse because he will have to have pain medication administered. And his leg is in a cast that makes his leg protrude straight out when in the wheelchair. You can only move him when the halls of the school are clear, not when all the students are switching classes. Otherwise, somehow his leg will get bumped, and it won't be pretty."

"Hmmm..."

"He's also on blood thinners."

She looked up at me. "Well, I don't see how that's a problem."

I took a deep breath, looked right back at her, and said very slowly and emphatically, "He is on *blood thinners*. What will you do if he, let's say, gets a cut and begins to bleed?"

At that point, she finally got the picture and approved Jacob as homebound.

Jacob's homebound teacher came by twice a week. She was wonderful with him. He was able to keep up with his schoolwork and maintain his grades.

During his recovery, we had numerous appointments with Dr. Monroe. We always scheduled an early appointment, so the trek to the doctor's office began in the dark hours of the morning. Jacob and I could watch the sun rise as we made our way to the medical center. During those drives I listened to Christian radio. Almost without fail, we heard the song "Stronger" by Mandisa.

The lyrics to this song became an anthem to me and to Jacob through this time of healing:

> When the waves are taking you under, hold on just a little bit longer
> He knows that this is gonna make you stronger, stronger
> The pain ain't gonna last forever, and things can only get better
> Believe me, this is gonna make you stronger.*

---

* Mandisa, "Stronger," recorded April 2011, track 1 on *What If We Were Real*, Capitol CMG Publishing.

"The pain ain't gonna last forever"—that was such an incredible promise. Once again I knew Jacob's struggle indeed was only going to make him stronger and provide another opportunity to proclaim the goodness and faithfulness of God.

Eight weeks after the accident, the month of April arrived. Jacob's cast was removed, and he began physical therapy. It was time to return to school. I loaded up his wheelchair every morning and got him into the school. He took it from there. After the wheelchair came the walker. Because of the coordination issues caused by Asperger's syndrome, Jacob wasn't able to master crutches, so he used the walker. He relied on the walker for about ten days, and then he graduated to a cane.

Physical therapy continued throughout July until eventually Jacob's leg was strong enough to resume normal activity.

Wrapping up Junior High

Despite the traumatic events of his seventh-grade year, everything went well during the remainder of junior high. We discovered in junior high that exceedingly loud noises bothered Jacob. The school held several pep rallies during the year in the gym. The band played, and all the students yelled and cheered. Jacob quickly recognized that it was too much for him to handle and asked to be removed to a quieter area. The school staff was happy to comply and always provided an alternative location for Jacob during pep rallies.

Throughout middle school and junior high, Jacob continued to attend weekly behavior group meetings.

The only issue we continued to have was his inability to get unstuck when he didn't understand an assignment. Spontaneous writing assignments were especially difficult for him. He is a great writer, but when a teacher instructed the class to write a paper or essay, he froze. Just as there were too many library books to choose from years ago, there were now too many possible topics for him to settle on one.

As a musician, I noticed over the years that Jacob had an amazing ear for music. He could sing a cappella and never veer off pitch. He could sing difficult intervals with ease, and I taught him to sing harmony with me. Since I am an instrumentalist and former band director, I encouraged him to join band in sixth grade, but he knew the noise level would be too much for him to handle. I was tempted to continue to pressure him to at least try band, but I was learning to let Jacob make his own decisions and backed off.

Since I am a piano teacher, I asked Jacob one day if he would like to learn to play the piano.

He looked at me very seriously and replied, "I'm not sure. I don't know how to play the piano."

I laughed. Good old Asperger's syndrome making itself known again—that fear of the unknown causing hesitation and uncertainty.

"Of course you don't know how to play the piano," I said. "That's the point of taking lessons."

"Oh, yes," he answered. "That's true."

He kindly placated me and gave it a good try, but in the end, he had no interest in the piano.

He joined the choir in eighth grade with some concern about the sound, but it was a great fit for him, and he enjoyed the class a lot.

High School Begins

With junior high successfully completed, it was time for high school. Jacob decided to attend a brand new high school starting with his freshman year. Students there could enroll in typical high school courses but were also offered college classes on the same campus. Jacob met with the counselor before the school year began and planned out his courses and his track of study for the next four years.

A week before school began, he attended the required freshman orientation.

Just a few days prior to the orientation, Jacob asked, "Mom, what's going to be happening at the orientation?"

Looking up from the meal I was cooking, I replied, "I'm not sure. They'll probably just go over some rules and stuff."

A few hours later, it hit me—hard. I had seen "the look." It had been so long that I had forgotten. Jacob was going to walk into a huge, two-story, brand new school with hundreds of kids he'd never met before to spend four hours doing, well, who knew? And I had pretty much just blown off his concerns.

I called him back downstairs and anxiously waited as he plodded down the steps.

"You were asking about orientation? Well, I know they're going to have a scavenger hunt, so you need a

QR reader app on your phone. They'll also go over first-day procedures. Other than that, I'm not certain what will happen, but if you have any questions, you can ask someone. Okay? Can you handle that?"

"Sure," he replied and headed back up the stairs.

I sat on the couch and placed my head in my hands. *How could I have forgotten? Why did I not remember his anxiety over change and new things? Wait! This is a good thing!*

Good? you ask. How can that be?

Because it had been such a long time since this was an issue that it didn't even register. That's called progress.

And it gets even better.

When I picked Jacob up from orientation a few days later and asked him how it went, he simply replied, "Boring."

"Did you have any questions?"

"Yeah. When I got to the cafeteria, I didn't know what line to stand in, so I went and asked someone."

He said it as if it was no big deal, and for him, it wasn't. But for me—well, the "Hallelujah Chorus" was exploding in my brain. I had lived through too many times when something as simple as not knowing which line to stand in would have caused a meltdown, at the least. And here we were. Not anymore.

When the new school year began, I stood in the driveway and watched as Jacob climbed into the car with Riley, who was driving. This was the first time ever that I wasn't the one to take him to the first day of his school year.

I was nervous because he had to go in the school, pick up his schedule, and then find all his classes. I watched the clock all day, and as soon as Jacob walked in the front door that afternoon, I pounced and said, "How was it? How did it go?"

"Great." And that was it.

I'm So Over That

One morning during his freshman year, Jacob texted me shortly after he left to inform me he had left his pencil bag at home. Knowing that would leave him without any pens or pencils to use during the day, I frantically tried to think of a way to deliver it to him immediately. The problem was that I had to drive Keaton to junior high, and his school started much later. By the time I could get the pencil bag delivered, Jacob would be well into his second class period.

I envisioned every possible, awful scenario in my fertile imagination. I could see Jacob sitting in class, frozen in a shutdown because the teacher had uttered those horrifying words, "Get out your pencil." I knew he wouldn't ask a friend to borrow one because, well, that's what kids with Asperger's syndrome do—or don't do. I even frantically attempted to phone his resource teacher, Mrs. Granger, so she could intervene, but she was unavailable.

Finally, an hour later, I pulled up in front of the school, threw my car in park, and literally ran inside. I breathlessly entered the main office. The receptionist looked up, noticed my flushed face and crazy hair, and still was able to calmly ask, "May I help you?"

I recanted in feverish detail the problem, detailing all my concerns and fears with apocalyptic intensity. She patiently awaited the end of my diatribe and said, "I'll see that he gets it."

That was it? I stood there too long, toying with the idea of rushing past the security guard, making my way upstairs, and screaming, "Jacob, I brought your pencil bag!" But instead, I turned around and made my way back to the car.

I'm ashamed to admit that I worried about it all day long.

When Jacob walked in the door from school, the first thing I said was, "Jacob, did you get your pencil bag?"

"Yes, I did. Thanks for bringing it."

I waited. Nothing else? No tales of angst? "Jacob, I was really worried. I knew you were sitting there in class without a pencil having a shutdown. I even tried to call Mrs. Granger to ask for her help."

Jacob stopped what he was doing and looked at me.

"Mom, I'm *so* over that."

He turned and walked upstairs.

I smiled and muttered to myself, "Yes, yes, you are!" I should have trusted in that very fact.

Leading the ARD Meeting

During Jacob's freshman year, I was the last to arrive to his annual ARD meeting. As I walked in and took my place, I glanced around at the high school staff seated around the large conference table. My attention was immediately drawn to the young man seated at the head of the table — my son Jacob.

Typically, one of the special education specialists served as the facilitator, but since Jacob was 15, the law required him to lead the meeting.

Jacob read from a prepared agenda and asked everyone to introduce themselves. He then continued down the list, addressing each item listed. He was funny and insightful. He listened, gave input, and answered questions.

I chuckled to myself as Jacob informed his math teacher, who was present at the meeting, that her class was too noisy and that she had seated him between the two most talkative students.

As the group went over Jacob's schedule for the upcoming school year, there was a big decision on course selection that he needed to make. Much to my surprise, Jacob had studied the schedule before the meeting and was able to easily inform the counselor which courses he had selected.

Oh, and can I mention that the staff in the ARD meeting commented on Jacob's impressive test scores? And let's not forget that the teachers in attendance bragged on what a great kid he was, adding that they wished they had a class full of students just like him. And I'd be remiss if I didn't include their comments on how polite, kind, and funny Jacob was.

I couldn't help but recall how I struggled with having Jacob classified as special ed when he was first diagnosed. My knee-jerk reaction was to not allow the school to attach that label to him. I admit it. I was ashamed. Pure selfishness and vanity were standing in the way of my child receiving the help he needed.

Now, as I sat in that conference and watched Jacob take the lead in his ARD meeting, I couldn't have been more proud. Whenever Jacob was referred to as being classified on the autism spectrum or having Asperger's syndrome, I would watch him to see if he would wince with embarrassment or shame. Nope. He took it all in stride. He had made the choice a long time ago to face Asperger's syndrome head on and emerge victorious.

Driving Lessons

We enrolled Jacob in driver's education the summer between his ninth and tenth grade years. In Texas, parents are required to give six months of behind-the-wheel instruction before a sixteen-year-old can receive his or her license. Dariel and I started working with Jacob as soon as all his driver's education requirements were completed, but we knew when his sixteenth birthday rolled around that he wasn't ready.

We were partly to blame because our own responsibilities had restricted the amount of time we could spend with Jacob driving under our instruction. But honestly, we knew it was not the right time. He needed more experience.

We kept working with him, and in May of his junior year, he passed his driving test and became a legal, licensed driver. Dariel purchased a new car for himself and gave Jacob his used 2007 Toyota Corolla. Jacob didn't care that it had more than 100,000 miles on it. He had his own car.

About a week after Jacob received his license, I was driving Keaton home from school when we turned the corner into our subdivision and saw Jacob's Corolla, a truck I had never seen, and two police cars. Wondering why Jacob hadn't called me about whatever was happening, I parked close to the Corolla and looked down at my phone. Jacob had called, but my phone was on vibrate, and I hadn't heard it.

My heart stopped. Keaton and I got out of my car and hurried over to Jacob, who was visibly upset.

"Jacob, what happened?"

"I hit that freaking (but he didn't say freaking) truck!"

"Jacob, we don't use that kind of language. Tell me what happened."

Jacob was trying to get by on the left side of the truck at an intersection on the way home from school. He misjudged the distance, and his side view mirror scratched the truck. He realized immediately what had happened, but the road he turned onto was a major thoroughfare with nowhere to pull over until the entrance to our subdivision. The woman driving the truck he scraped followed him and called the police, thinking Jacob was attempting to flee the scene.

Jacob handed over his driver's license and insurance card to one of the policemen as the officer berated him for not pulling over immediately after the accident.

I didn't want to use Asperger's syndrome as an excuse. I did not. But I did.

"Officer, Jacob has Asperger's syndrome, which can cause extreme anxiety in unknown situations. He drove here because that's what he knew. Our neighborhood is familiar to him."

"Well, that's not right. I could arrest him for fleeing the scene. There were plenty of places he could have pulled over."

No, there weren't. I drove that stretch of road at least twice a day, six days a week, and I could not think of one place where I would have been comfortable stopping my car. But in that moment, I thought it was best just to keep my mouth shut.

I wanted to say, *Go ahead. Arrest him. I'll get a lawyer and you won't know what hit you. You're threatening to take a 17-year-old young man with Asperger's syndrome into custody.* But a cooler head prevailed. I just nodded and said, "Yes, sir."

As the police officer was completing his accident report, I went back over to Jacob.

"Jacob, why were you using the 'f' word? We don't say that word ever in our home."

He answered, "I know it's not a good word, but I thought it was appropriate for this situation."

Despite the circumstances, I wanted to laugh. That was a classic Asperger's syndrome response.

Miraculously, there was only minor damage to the woman's truck, which we gladly paid for. She was incredibly kind and understanding.

Jacob's side view mirror was ripped off, and there was damage to the passenger door, but we got it taken care of the next day at minimal cost. The Corolla isn't very pretty anymore, but it's paid off, repaired, and able to transport Jacob wherever he needs to go.

As frightening as it was for Dariel and me to let Jacob get behind the wheel again, we knew we had to. We didn't want Jacob's fear to overwhelm him. It was important to get him driving again. As soon as we got his car back from the auto shop, Jacob was driving himself once again to and from school and church.

Making a Difference

After Jacob's freshman year, his coach at Behavior Plus had asked him to attend an extra class once a week, not as a participant but as a student coach. Jacob had the opportunity to help kids who were walking the path he had already gone down. We considered it such an honor.

The following year, Jacob decided he didn't want to attend behavior group anymore. He had been in the program so long that he found the majority of the information repetitive. The timing of his decision was good since our family had moved to the other side of town. The coaches at Behavior Plus still check in with him from time to time and let him know they'd love to have him return.

In the fall semester of Jacob's sophomore year in high school, he enrolled in a college speech class. After exchanging several emails and phone calls with his professor, Dariel and I decided he should drop the class. Jacob simply couldn't get up in front of the class to make a speech, and his grade was suffering.

What a difference a teacher can make! In the spring semester, Jacob signed up for speech again, but this time with a different teacher. He sailed through the course with no problems. The teacher emailed me halfway through the semester to let me know how proud she was of Jacob. He had received the highest grade in the class on two of his speeches. She was also impressed that when a student in the class was too fearful to stand and give his speech, Jacob volunteered to go to the front of the class with him and help him deliver it successfully.

Wow! My Jacob? The same Jacob that wouldn't give a speech the previous semester? I was so proud. And the next school year, when he was a junior, he wrote a very special essay for his English class. I had no idea he was going to write on the subject he chose. I cry every time I read it. Let me share it with you.

> *Everyone has a trait or characteristic that makes them unique; something they believe they would be incomplete without. Generally speaking, these life-defining traits are typically positive, such as intelligence or a natural singing ability. However, in the case of myself, my life-defining trait is my Asperger's syndrome, and I certainly would not be where I am without it. My strange behavior was very noticeable as a child. As a baby, I had a knack for throwing things across the room to see how far they would go, and I hated having to wear socks and shoes. But you wouldn't question this type of behavior, would you? Babies are weird, so they have weird behaviors. I wouldn't question a baby who likes to throw things across a room, personally. However, as I got older, my behavior became more "problematic." Whenever I didn't understand how to do something or I got frustrated, which happened quite often, I would "shut down" and refuse to speak to anyone about the problem, or anyone in general. At this time, I was prone to frequent ear infections, and I would never say anything about them. I would sit there, totally silent, until my parents could visibly tell I had an ear infection. Even worse still, this bad habit got me expelled during first grade. Eventually, we came to understand the problem. What had originally been thought as behavioral*

problems turned out to be Asperger's syndrome, and everything began to make sense. I began to go to behavior counseling and stayed there for several years. It's not like all of my problems would instantly fade; I was as problematic in counseling as I was outside of counseling. The only difference now was that I was actually learning how to control myself. I slowly began to understand figurative language and nonverbal social cues, both of which I struggled with beforehand. I learned how to deal with change, and most importantly, I learned how to ask questions. Certainly, I've benefited from Asperger's syndrome more than I've suffered. If it weren't for Asperger's, I wouldn't have gone to behavior counseling to learn the social skills I needed to hold conversation. If it weren't for Asperger's, I wouldn't have gone to behavior counseling to learn how to ask questions whenever I needed help, and how to talk about my problems instead of having shutdowns. As bad as Asperger's syndrome sounds at first, I don't ever think of it as a curse. I always think of it as a blessing.

During the summer before his senior year, Jacob started working part time at a local fast food restaurant. We opened a checking account for him at the same time. Watching him drive off to his job never got old. I was in awe. If you had told me we'd be here ten years ago when I was walking into that elementary school listening as my child's screams filled the halls, I would have never believed you. Not one bit.

Graduation and Beyond

On May 26, 2017, Jacob walked across the stage to receive his high school diploma. His brothers, parents, paternal grandparents, and aunt were all there to cheer him on.

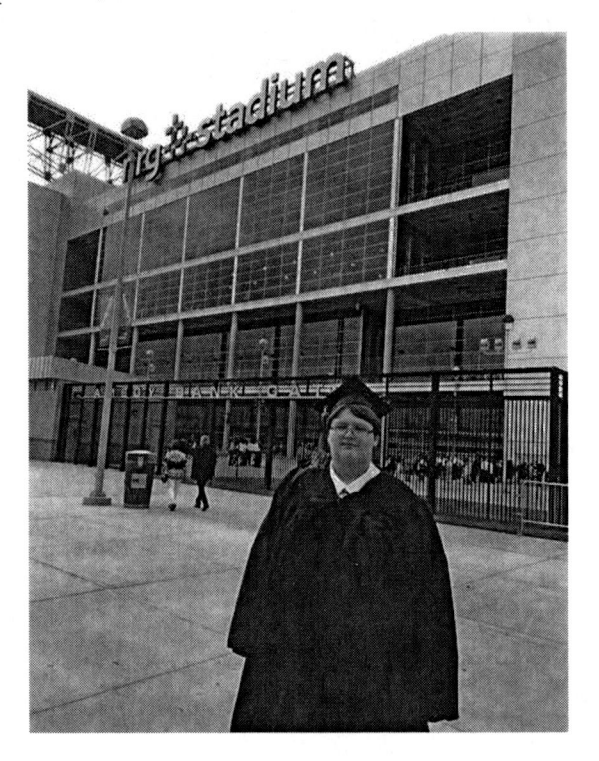

As we waited in the huge arena for the graduation to begin, I was overcome with emotion as I reflected on how far we'd traveled to be there in that moment, only minutes away from Jacob crossing the finish line of his public school education. Dariel and I vividly recalled every minute of those first few months of anguish when Jacob was initially diagnosed and enrolled in Whispering Pines Elementary School. All the memories, positive and negative, only served to make Jacob's special day that much sweeter.

Jacob was scheduled to graduate not only with his high school diploma but also with his associate's degree from a local community college. Jacob had completed more than 30 hours of college courses, but he was not able to complete all his classes before graduation, so he didn't receive the associate's degree.

After graduation, Jacob enrolled in summer school to take the last two classes required for the two-year associate's degree. I would be remiss if I didn't admit that his delay in completing the degree is due in part to his shutdowns. Jacob often does not complete assignments because he doesn't understand what to do. And even though he knows to ask for help, he chooses not to, and the work doesn't get done or a penalty is applied when it's turned in past the due date. We're trying desperately to allow Jacob to handle all of this with the professors. When he works for his bachelor's degree, it needs to be all him and not Mom and Dad to the rescue. It's one of the most difficult things we've ever done.

I must admit that I was very disappointed when Jacob passed only one of the two remaining courses he took in the summer at the community college, and thus he will not receive the associate's degree. He has been accepted at a local four-year university where the majority of his community college credits will be transferred, but I very much wanted him to receive that degree.

When Jacob informed me that he had not passed the last class, I was initially angry but successfully kept that in control. I could tell immediately that he was already beating himself up for not passing, and I didn't want to add to that. I expressed my disappointment to him but made the conscious decision to be happy that he had successfully completed many college hours that would be transferred to the new school.

The course Jacob failed that summer was an online course. It was the second online course he didn't pass. We've learned that online is not the best learning atmosphere for him.

Even with everything I've learned these last twelve school years, even with all the stories I've shared to this point, I must confess that I'm struggling once again. The college Jacob will attend to earn his bachelor's degree is about a forty-five-minute drive from our house through a densely populated area with many turns, traffic lights, and tons of traffic. Jacob has attended orientation there the past couple of weeks and taken a test required prior to admittance. Dariel and I allowed him to drive the route but with us in a car alongside him. He's not quite comfortable with how to get to the college on his own, and in an attempt to keep it real, Dariel and I are both scared to death of Jacob driving that far by himself and through so much traffic. Will we allow him do it? Yes, but as is the case through much of this journey, it's not going to be easy.

The Journey Is the Reward

As I mentioned earlier, for every step forward, we sometimes take one step back. But isn't that life in a nutshell? Nothing is perfect all the time. Things rarely go as we hope. From the defeats, we learn to pick ourselves up and try again. It's the ultimate Do Over.

I think this whole experience is best summarized in this statement: "The journey is the true reward because it is in the process that we develop the Christ-likeness we need to walk in the promises he has given us."[*] The *journey* is the reward.

Jacob is on this journey. By allowing him to struggle, he becomes stronger. By allowing him to fail, he becomes more determined to prevail and enjoys success that much more. By allowing him to fall down, he is humbled when he has to ask for help to stand up and walk.

It's also my huge reward as I walk beside Jacob. I have become stronger in the struggle. I have failed with Jacob so many times that it's made me a better person and a better parent. And with each success Jacob enjoys, I revel in the faithfulness and love of my amazing God.

---

[*] Pastor Tom Allen (class notes, Crosspoint Church, Pearland, TX, Fall, 2011).

8

SPEAK LIFE

God is our merciful Father and the source of all comfort. He comforts us in all our troubles so that we can comfort others. When they are troubled, we will be able to give them the same comfort God has given us.

—2 Corinthians 1:3–4 (NLT)

Recently, while attending orientation at the four-year college where Jacob will complete his bachelor's degree, the director of Disability Services for the campus informed us that over the last two years, the college has seen a 600 percent increase in freshmen diagnosed on the autism spectrum. That is a very difficult statistic for me to wrap my brain around.

But it helps me understand the numerous people I've encountered from all walks of life who've faced many of the same challenges my family went through with Jacob and also why so many are eager to know what we learned along the way.

There is often a desperation in the questions people ask me as they desire, just as my family did so many years ago, to not only understand Asperger's syndrome but also to learn how to overcome it.

Years ago, after Jacob was settled in at Whispering Pines Elementary School, I began working part time for the worship pastor of our church. Since Community Christian Academy, the private school, and the church were located in the same building, I frequently had interaction with the school staff.

One day, Mrs. Sanders, the kindergarten teacher I confronted with the letter from the psychiatrist, sought me out in my office.

"Julie, I have a student in my class that I'd like you to come and observe. His behavior reminds me so much of Jacob's, and I want to see what you think. I'm considering talking to his parents about Asperger's syndrome, but I'd like your input first."

God knows just where to get me every time. I was both honored and humbled that she would come to me. "Mrs. Sanders, I'm not a doctor, so I wouldn't be able to tell you with any certainty. If you think Asperger's syndrome is a possibility, his parents need to have him tested."

"I realize that. I'm just curious to see what you think."

I agreed to take a look the next day and give my opinion.

Another time, a mother contacted me by email. She was curious about what kind of treatments were needed for children with Asperger's syndrome since her son had recently been diagnosed. I replied and shared with her the information we had received from the psychiatrist regarding Jacob. I sought to encourage her with details of how much improvement Jacob had made over time.

I'll never forget her reply: "I just want to do enough so my son doesn't bother my husband anymore."

Just enough? I could not believe she said that. The child needed to be given the tools to succeed and make the most of his life. I was stunned.

Unfortunately, that exchange wouldn't be the last of its kind. I've spoken to many more people along the way who expressed the very same sentiment.

Often when Jacob was attending his weekly group at Behavior Plus, I spent time talking with Mrs. Kling. I brought up women I had exchanged emails with and bemoaned the fact that so many were unwilling to put in the work. Mrs. Kling said that she was faced with that same situation repeatedly at Behavior Plus. She said the majority of parents spend large amounts of money paying for the group sessions, drop their child off for the weekly meetings, and then do nothing at home to follow through.

That disturbing fact still causes me great sadness.

Would Dariel and I rather have been doing other things? You bet! Was it difficult? More than words on a page can adequately express. Is Jacob worth it? Absolutely. Consistency, determination, and faith yielded incredible results.

Often, I excitedly emailed Mrs. Kling or told her in person of Jacob's newest accomplishment. She told me that when she traveled as a guest speaker for various workshops and conferences, she frequently shared with her audience what she called "Jacob stories." Mrs. Kling had been there from the beginning, and it was her delight to tell others about what could be accomplished. Once again, Jacob was impacting people around him, many of whom he would never meet.

One evening at Behavior Plus, when I was filling in Mrs. Kling on Jacob's latest achievement, she looked at me and said, "You should write a book." I was startled because for almost a year I had felt God urging me to author a book about our journey with Jacob. I had not expressed that to anyone, not even my husband. And there it was, God affirming through this exceptional woman what he had laid on my heart many months ago.

I often remember the moment when my frightened six-year-old boy came to me and asked why he was being shuttled from one doctor to another. Twelve years later, those words God gave me to speak hope into that young heart are truer than ever: "Jacob, one day you're going to come out on the other side of this with an amazing testimony. God is going to use you to help others."

God has taught me so many things through this journey.

I learned that he wants me to seek him for everything (Matt. 6:33).

I learned that parenting isn't for cowards, and because of everything that has transpired, I've become a better mother, wife, teacher, and person (Rom. 8:28).

I learned that God gives us family for a reason. Jacob has been loved in every situation, cheered for every success, and encouraged by all (Eccles. 4:9–12).

I learned that God does not want us to exist in a vacuum. He desires that we seek help. Where would Jacob be today without the wonderful coaches from Behavior Plus who poured their lives into his? And where would we be as a family without our church community of friends and pastors who prayed faithfully for us and impacted Jacob's life on so many levels (Gal. 6:2)?

I've learned that having a special needs child doesn't make me a failure as a mother. I didn't do anything wrong, and I'm not being punished. I made the choice—and it *was* a choice—to see this experience not as a curse but as a huge gift (James 1:17).

And most importantly, I've learned that we love and serve a God who is so much bigger than we can begin to imagine. He is my strength, my joy, my rock, and my provider (Phil. 4:13).

With every success story I've shared about Jacob, I would ask you to remember that none of it came easily. But then, the best things in life never do.

EPILOGUE

"Mom, why did God give me Asperger's?"
That's the question of a lifetime, isn't it? When Dariel returned home from work, we sat Jacob down and did our best to provide him with a Bible-based answer that could be easily understood by a nine-year-old.

"Jacob," Dariel began, "do you remember the story from the book of Genesis that tells how sin entered the world through Adam and Eve in the garden?"

He nodded.

"When God created the world, everything was perfect. Adam and Eve had perfect bodies that would never get sick or hungry because there was no sin."

We were good so far.

"Well, God had provided Adam and Eve with everything they needed, but they thought they knew better than God. So they made the choice to disobey God's command, and sin entered the world. And because sin came into the world, people weren't perfect anymore. They could get sick and experience pain and hunger. Babies were born sometimes with really bad illnesses or other problems. It's no one's fault, and it isn't their parents' fault. It's just what happens when we live in a world with sin."

"So God did not *give* you Asperger's syndrome," I said. "It exists in the world because of sin. Doctors believe it may be passed down in families, so if that's true, someone in my family or Daddy's family may have had Asperger's syndrome and passed it on to you."

"Who had it?" he asked.

"Well, again, if it is passed down in families, we don't know. It's still such a new discovery that it would have gone unrecognized and untreated because no none knew anything about Asperger's syndrome back then."

"But one day, when we are living with Jesus in heaven," Dariel said, "we will all have new, perfect bodies."

He perked up. "So you mean I'm going to get a new body one day when I go to heaven?"

"Yes, you will. All Christians will."

"And I won't have Asperger's, and I can maybe fly?" That sense of humor.

"I'm not sure about that last one," Dariel responded, "but yes, no more Asperger's."

"That's awesome!" Jacob declared.

My husband and I aren't anything special. As I hope I have demonstrated, we've had our share of failures. We've struggled with doubt. We've wallowed at times in self-pity and demanded answers from God in moments of anger.

In great humility and with overwhelming gratitude, I recognize the incredible gift God entrusted to my husband and me when he knit Jacob together in my womb. What a special, special child God gave us to raise.

If I can offer any advice to parents, it's this. Be your children's strength when they can't be strong. Be their hope when they're disappointed and discouraged. Be their biggest cheerleader when they get it right. And be their advocate and fight for what they need to make it in this world and be successful. Give them your time, and don't settle for just enough to get by.

My greatest prayer when I started this book was that I would hold nothing back. My desire was to share the stories that made me laugh, the defeats and challenges that made me cry, the victories that made me stand up and cheer, and the trials that brought me to my knees.

Why? Because early on in this journey, I made the decision to give it all to God—all the glory, all the hope for the future, all the pain, and all the heartache. I laid it at his feet and said, "I can't do this; I do not want to do this without You. Be my strength in my overwhelming weakness."

We're not done. As I shared earlier, Jacob is starting college and looks forward to a career, living on his own, getting married, and starting a family.

God has only begun his work in my son. I'm excited to see what other incredible "Jacob stories" we'll someday share with others to encourage, inspire, and bring glory to God.

Family - Jacob at age 2

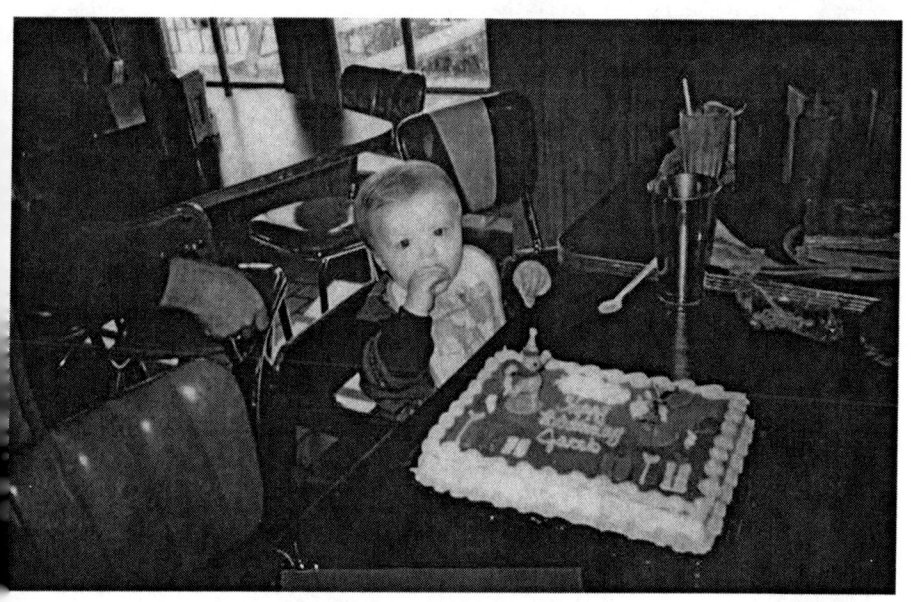

Jacob's 1st birthday

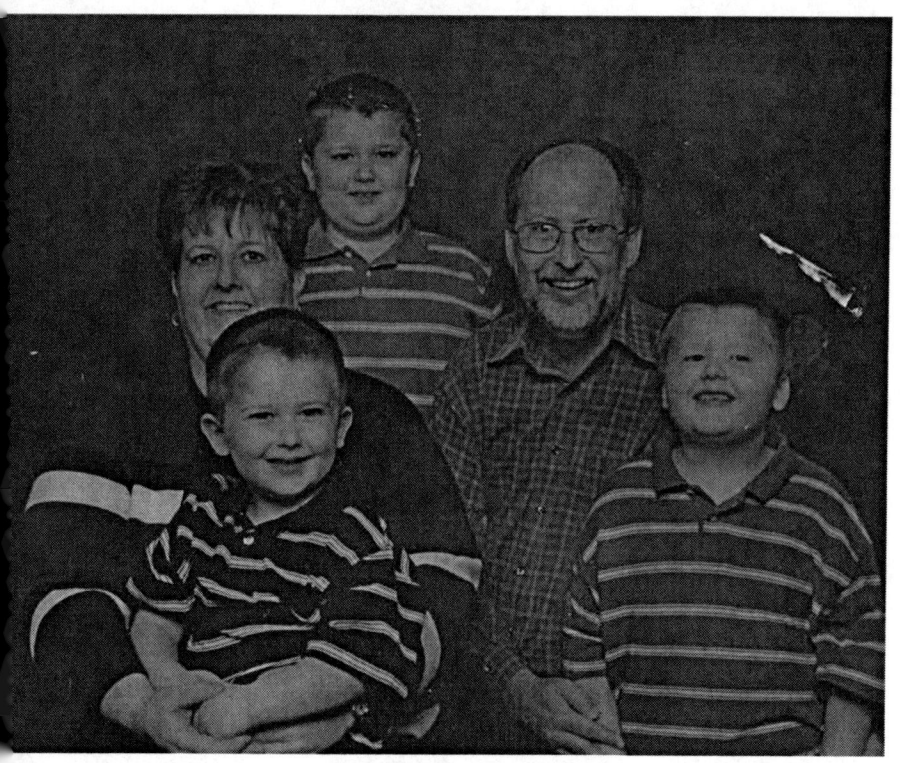

Family - Jacob at age 6

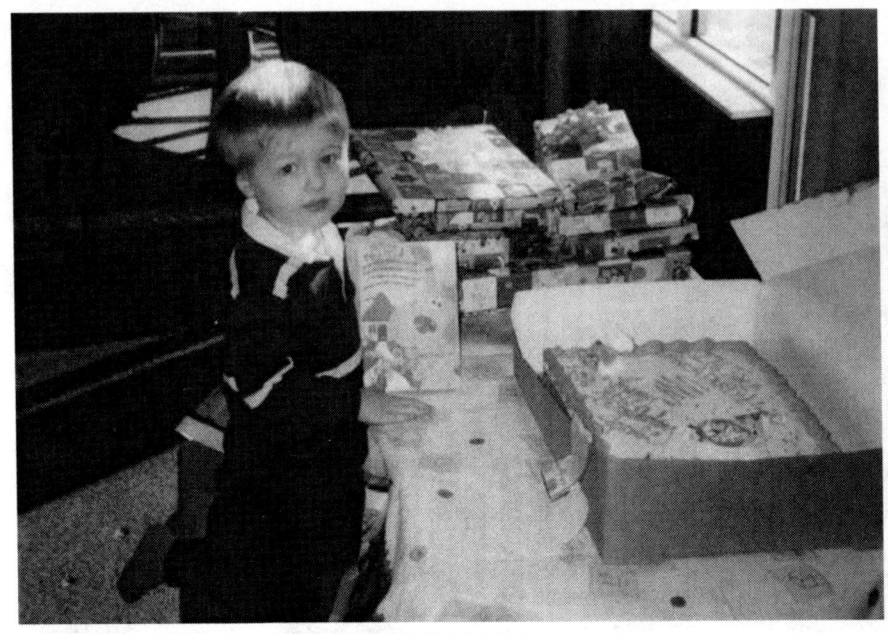

Jacob's 3rd birthday

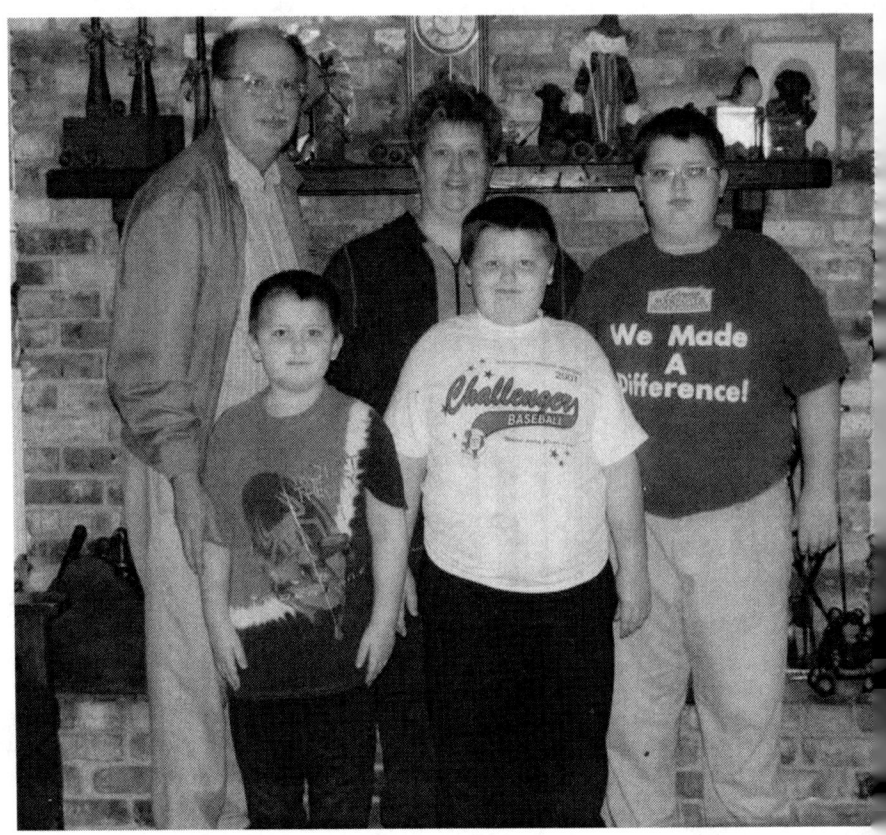

Family - Jacob at age 7

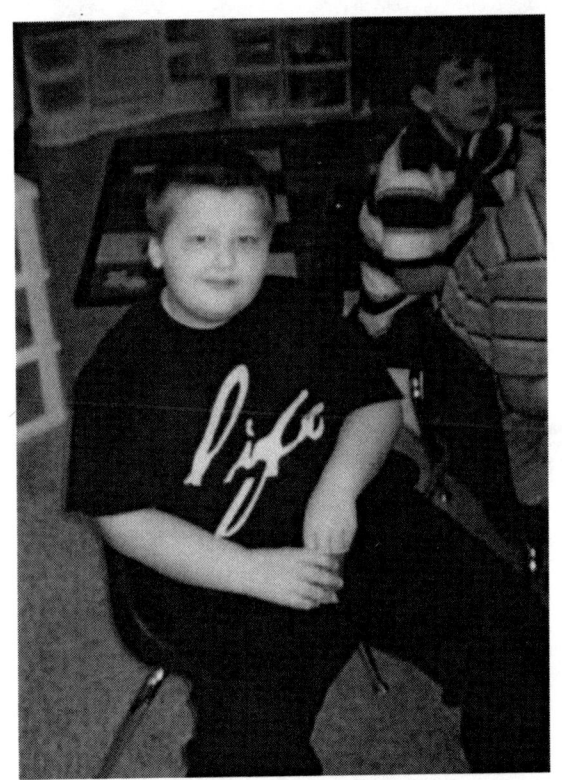

Jacob - 2nd grade

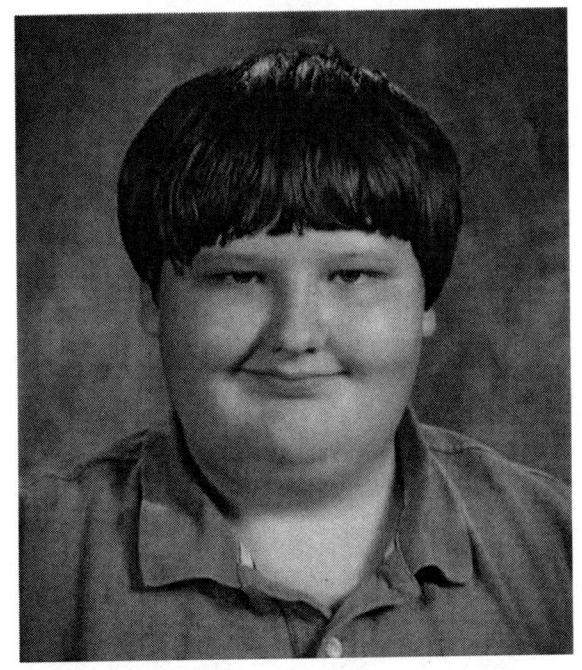

Jacob - 5th grade

CPSIA information can be obtained
at www.ICGtesting.com
Printed in the USA
FFOW01n2340080418
46190896-47455FF